Happy-Go-Yoga

Happy-Go-Yoga

Simple Poses to Relieve Pain, Reduce Stress, and Add Joy

Christine Chen

Illustrations by Cody Shipman

GRAND CENTRAL
Life & Style
NEW YORK · BOSTON

Grand Central Life & Style

Hachette Book Group

1290 Avenue of the Americas

New York, NY 10104

www.HachetteBookGroup.com

Printed in the United States of America

RRD-C

First Edition: March 2015

10 9 8 7 6 5 4 3 2 1

Grand Central Life & Style is an imprint of Grand Central Publishing.

The Grand Central Life & Style name and logo are trademarks of Hachette Book Group, Inc.

The Hachette Speakers Bureau provides a wide range of authors for speaking events. To find out more, go to www.hachettespeakersbureau.com or call (866) 376-6591.

The publisher is not responsible for websites (or their content) that are not owned by the publisher.

Library of Congress Cataloging-in-Publication Data

Chen, Christine.
    Happy-go-yoga : simple poses to relive pain, reduce stress, and add joy / Christine Chen. — First edition.
        pages cm
    Includes bibliographical references and index.
    ISBN 978-1-4555-8193-1 (pbk.) — ISBN 978-1-4555-8194-8 (ebook)   1. Hatha yoga—Therapeutic use.
2. Posture.   3. Exercise therapy.   4. Paint—Treatment.   I. Title.
    RA781.7.C4724 2015
    613.7'046—dc23
                                        2014020874

I dedicate this book to everyone who wants to feel better and be happier.

table of contents

foreword

Why Happy-Go-Yoga?

by Paul J. Christo, MD

introduction

How I Got Happy: The Author's Story

chapter one

Who, Why, and How to Happy-Go-Yoga

chapter two

Travel Buddies

**Relief for your back, body, and mind
during long flights and challenging commutes**

Eagle Perch ▪ Eagle Twist ▪ Bird's Eye ▪ Bird of Prey ▪ Hang Time
Grounded in a Good Way ▪ Reach for the Moon
Walk Your Puppies ▪ Pray to the Seat Pocket ▪ Smooth Landing

Why Happy-Go-Yoga?

Paul J. Christo, MD

Host of Aches and Gains *and Associate Professor,*
Division of Pain Medicine, Johns Hopkins University School of Medicine

When Christine decided to embark on writing a book on yoga that would encourage body movement for good health, stress reduction, and pain relief, I was excited. Our modern lifestyle has significantly reduced natural movement and replaced it with inaction. We sit in front of computers for hours each day. We sit in cars, trains, buses, or airplanes en route to meetings, our job, or even leisure activities. At night, we sit in plush chairs or lie on comfortable couches to watch our favorite reality TV shows.

Unfortunately, all of this sedentary time has led to unfavorable health outcomes. More of us are obese, have heart disease, suffer from diabetes, and constantly strain the joints of our spines and limbs. We're designed to move, yet we're mostly immobile. The benefits of exercise are numerous, but most important, it's the fundamental step toward feeling better.

Evidence of the growing value of complementary and alternative medicine (CAM) and therapies like yoga for reaching optimal health and healing is steadily increasing. A 2007 National Health Interview Survey reported that more than 38 percent of American adults and almost 12 percent of children used some type of CAM therapy during the previous year. In fact, pain is among the most common reasons for seeking CAM treatments and specifically for easing lower-back pain.

It's easy to understand why more of my own pain patients are feeling the positive effects of CAM treatments, and especially yoga. As a form of exercise and moving meditation, yoga offers them pain relief, improves their mood and body mass index, and helps them reduce risk factors associated with chronic diseases. Patients tell me that the deep stretching combined with relaxation and the deep and rhythmic breathing of yoga promotes well-being and comfort. It makes them feel better, more alive, and more able to withstand the stresses of daily life.

Today, we're learning more about the effects on the body of slow and deep breathing. Interestingly, some studies tell us that slow breathing reduces pain, and some experts feel that slow, deep breathing suppresses the sympathetic nervous system (fight or flight response), which in turn influences how pain is processed in the nervous system.

If you look at the evidence for yoga's effects on pain, you'll see that the practice allows patients to better cope with the biological, psychological, and social dimensions of having persistent pain. This is critical because pain can take over your life and make you feel like you're a prisoner. Yoga offers a way out through gentle exercise and a refreshing relaxation. I've seen benefits in patients with arthritis in easing tender and swollen joints. And I've seen yoga help patients with fibromyalgia lessen their pain and fatigue and elevate their mood and ability to cope. And I've heard from patients that they feel less stressed, more resilient, and less injury-prone.

Yoga is low risk, low cost, and well tolerated. This is a perfect trio for my own patients who may be afraid of worsening their pain or who may have limited finances. Yoga can be practiced in class or even at home. Even simple exercises can be taught in the doctor's office for those too injured or otherwise unable to take classes. Researchers are currently studying the effects of yoga on older adults specifically because of its global benefit to health and balance.

I mentioned initially that I was excited, and now you can understand the reason. *Happy-Go-Yoga* helps you take that first step toward mobilizing your body and mind. As an experienced yoga instructor, Christine Chen has written a smart, fun, and easy guide for healthy living. Yoga offers you the potential to improve your life, feel better, and regain a sense of wellness.

As a pain specialist who's seen many patients freed from their discomfort, I'm enthusiastic about the promise of CAM treatments, and especially yoga. I hope that in reading Christine's book, you're able to awaken a new potential to take care of yourself, overcome any medical limitations, and achieve what you want in life.

Happy-Go-Yoga

How I Got Happy: The Author's Story

I went to my first yoga class in 1999 to tackle stress and back pain. At the time I was a news anchor and reporter, and I was unable to sit at the news desk or stand for a live report without experiencing shooting and/or throbbing pain. My high-octane life of constant deadlines, odd hours, lack of sleep, and weird working conditions manifested in two different spine conditions and high anxiety—bad news for a newsperson. Sometimes I would lie on the floor during commercial breaks just so I could feel enough relief to get up and muster a smile for the cameras despite the pain.

Every minute at work was filled with talk of disaster, crisis, controversy, and violence, all of which had taken a toll on my heart and my personal life. I had few coping skills for this level and type of stress, so, like many others in the industry, I became jaded, turned to cocktails, and held it all in—a recipe for toxicity. Three of my friends/coworkers with similar lifestyles were diagnosed with cancer in their mid-thirties, and one passed away a few years ago. Gratefully, I never got so sick that I was on life support, but certainly, I was not supporting my own health very well.

Because of my spine, my doctors banned me from nearly all the activities that helped me cope with stress, including the super-sweaty cardio workouts that also kept me slim and camera-ready. Doctors even instructed me to get in and out of a car a special way. Most nights I couldn't sleep without medication. Every part of my life was compromised by my health, and my health was being compromised by every part of my life—a terrible cycle that kept eroding my mind, body, and spirit. I felt like I was in a physical and emotional storm cloud every day. A single gal at the time, I was not a fun date. My soul was suffering, and I feared I would never find my soul mate. In a word, I was unhappy.

In the midst of an array of medical treatments for my spine problems, including anti-inflammatory spine injections, electro-stimulus, prescription drugs, acupuncture, and months of physical therapy, I tried yoga. I felt better physically, at first, just for short periods of time. I was skeptical about whether yoga would help me. Let's be honest; before, I had been stress busting by kickboxing, and this was the total opposite. But I found I was challenged physically by the poses and measurably calmer after each class. I was curious to know more. Doctors said that to "fix" my spine they would have to cut through the front of my neck for surgery. Even so, they could not guarantee total pain relief. Faced with that reality, I kept going to yoga.

I wavered between skeptic and willing student. I fit in as many classes as my schedule allowed and was fortunate to have knowledgeable and caring teachers. When I couldn't make it to class, I did pieces of the poses from class, and I did them everywhere. I stretched at the news desk during commercial breaks. I twisted in the corners of airports. I breathed deeply in traffic jams to relax. I meditated to cope with one chaotic situation after another. I can't recall exactly when things shifted, but yoga became part of my everyday life.

My spine specialists were skeptical, worried that yoga would hurt me rather than help me. They saw actual physical improvement, though, and they gave me a green light for more yoga. My body got stronger. My mind became calmer. I slept better, which gave my body a better shot at resting and repairing itself. Some modern medicine was needed to help treat me, but a pattern became clear to me: I could insert some kind of yoga in various moments of my day, and I would feel better. Guess what? I never had the spine surgery, and more than a decade after all these problems, I'm pretty much pain-free.

Today, an increasing number of medical studies support what I had discovered during my journey out of pain and stress: My mind helped my body feel better, and my body helped my mind feel better. What the yogis had experienced for thousands of years, I experienced in modern life. Without a doubt, I can say yoga was a major factor in transforming my health, and really, my life. Literally, my yoga practice was my medicine; it saved me—physically, emotionally, and spiritually. In my mid-forties now, I feel I am the healthiest version of me that's ever existed.

In a word, I got happy.

Deeply passionate about yoga's ability to transform, or at least just help people feel a little better each day, I decided to learn how to teach it. My students were delighted learning even the smallest things that made them feel better, and they wanted more for the times they couldn't come to class.

I spent the first twenty years of my career in the media, delivering news and information about the world via television and Web. Now, in this book, I feel I am broadcasting the most vital information I could possibly offer: an easy-to-understand, accessible way to help people feel better and be happier—regardless of level, age, gender, ethnicity, or life circumstances.

When I first started yoga, I could probably do only 20 percent of any class, if that. I had the following reactions: 1) I don't like this; 2) This isn't doing anything; 3) I don't feel anything; 4) This is a waste of my time; 5) I can't do these poses; 6) I don't like this teacher; and 7) I want to leave class. I hear a mix of those things from a lot of people who are new, have injuries, or have doubts. Believe me, I understand. I see people who are stressed, hurting, or struggling in some way, and it quickly takes me back to how I felt back then. Because I have been there, I can say with total authenticity to you and anyone, "You can feel better too! It'll take time. Try this. Keep doing it. It works."

While yoga was definitely my medicine, *Happy-Go-Yoga* is not a medical book, and I am not a doctor. This book is a collection of poses based on real yoga and real health information with a big dose of real life and a dash of whimsy. I have used these poses—fully or in pieces—again and again. I realize yoga can seem intimidating and mysterious, so I wanted to show that yoga can be very humble, simple, and fun! Back hurt from standing in line for so long?

There's a pose for that. Frustrated with your coworker? There's a pose for that. Emotionally drained from a family get-together? There's a pose for that. Hoping you can improve the communication in your relationship? There's a pose for that, too.

Yoga isn't about becoming a human pretzel, being vegan, or wearing trendy workout clothes to a green juice bar. It's a way of living and creating habits to live a life of less suffering and more peace and happiness. *Happy-Go-Yoga* is for all of us, even those who don't really "do yoga." It's the result of revelations in my own healing journey, hundreds of hours of teacher trainings, years of teaching students of all kinds, and my own ever-changing self-practice.

Back in the day, I had a go-to version of Pigeon Pose at the news desk for quick relief. A few years ago, when I moved to New York, the intensity of my new city had me spontaneously doing a version of Standing Half Moon on the subway to relieve my weary body from pounding the pavement. Intrigued, a woman standing on the subway next to me asked what I was doing. I explained; she started copying me and then started smiling right away. "This feels so good!" she said. Another woman, seated right next to us, was watching and listening to the whole thing. She stated, with the total conviction of a New Yorker, "You should write a book." And so I did. That moment became "Reach for the Moon" (p. 22).

I hope *Happy-Go-Yoga* helps you the way it helped me, my students, and the woman on the subway. You can feel better and be happier, too. It'll take time, but try this and keep doing it. It works.

chapter one

Who, Why, and How to Happy-Go-Yoga

Stress is being called the next big health crisis. More people today get back surgery than coronary bypasses or hip replacements. Study after study shows that a little bit of yoga goes a long way, and our efforts add up over time. UCLA researchers found that yoga helps alleviate pain and anxiety. At the University of Illinois, researchers found that yoga helps the brain work better, while Duke scientists concluded that yoga helps people sleep better. Ohio State researchers found that yoga reduces inflammation, and Taiwanese researchers found that yoga teachers have healthier spines.

Happy-Go-Yoga is my playful, witty take on traditional yoga, designed for people who don't have time for—or simply don't do—yoga. Even the biggest skeptics (and I was one of them) can do just a little at a time and start to experience the benefits. Our lives are more amped than ever before. We can't rely on just pills, doctor's visits, cocktails, or watching television to relax!

All you have to do is start with one *Happy-Go-Yoga* pose, just one, and see where that takes you. Do it to feel good, or do it to shift your mood. I'm telling you, it's fun, and you'll feel better.

How to Use *Happy-Go-Yoga*

If you're new to yoga, I recommend chatting with your doctor to sort out your own personal health situation first. Yoga is not a panacea or cure-all, but if you believe my story and many years' worth of stories, it helps on many levels.

You'll find that you can do just about every pose in *Happy-Go-Yoga*, and so can your mom, dad, grandma, grandpa, sister, brother, daughter, son, aunt, uncle, boss, coworker, BFF, bus driver, and neighbor. You might do Happy-Go-Yoga together. You might share a tip or two with someone you don't quite know as well (it's good karma)!

In the book's pages, each Happy-Go-Yoga pose is a mix of some very useful things: a potential situation in our daily lives, traditional yoga teachings, and brief nuggets of health knowledge gathered from my own experience, my studies, my teachers, many doctors, medical research, and health experts.

I suggest two easy ways to work Happy-Go-Yoga into your life:

Put Poses into Your Everyday Life

A bit of lower-back relief can make you a little less cranky toward everyone in the office (especially when the boss seems to be cranky for unknown reasons). A specific way of breathing can keep you from going crazy when there are just too many people around (story of my life in New York City). A type of hand gesture (not what you think) can help you invite a little more love into your life. A certain way of standing can inspire you to feel more confident when it counts (like right before a job interview). If you can relate to the real-life scenarios on each page, just follow the directions and illustrations.

Change How You Want to Feel—Anywhere, Anytime

Many of the poses do not need to be location- or situation-specific. If you know you need to feel less stressed quickly, you can look for the "De-stress" label throughout the book to find the right poses for you. Need relief from aches? Look for "Relieve" labels; there are poses for that. Need to be focused? Find the "Focus" label.

Take your pick:

- **De-stress:** Quickly reduce your anxiety, frustration, or fear
- **Relieve:** Give your brain and body relief from pain or discomfort
- **Relax:** Soothe, unwind, and feel comforted
- **Strengthen:** Firm and tone parts of the body
- **Empower:** Feel more confident and self-assured
- **Balance:** Feel steady physically, mentally, and spiritually
- **Calm:** Be mellow and unruffled by challenge
- **Love:** Be more affectionate and intimate with yourself and others
- **Brighten:** Get uplifted and more positive
- **Connect:** Link more authentically with yourself and others
- **Refresh:** Energize your body and awaken your mind
- **Focus:** Be less distracted and more present and productive
- **Inspire:** Encourage yourself and motivate others with your spirit

You can do all of the poses or some of them. You can share them with others and be the mini health hero in someone else's day. Some of the poses are not obvious body shapes, but things you do intentionally to cultivate a yogi state of mind. Remember: Some of the more subtle shifts are the most powerful.

And look for these on every pose page, too:

- **Tip:** An extra little bit of information that might help you in the pose
- **Bonus:** Another version that adds variety or a degree of difficulty to the pose
- **Note:** An FYI about things that could come up during the pose
- **Extra Karma:** Small things you can do to share your Happy-Go-Yoga moment

You'll get the most out of Happy-Go-Yoga if you're optimistic and open to the possibility that you can change your life by learning how to move and breathe consciously, one day at a time. Even if you're a skeptic, try being just a tiny bit open to the possibility. Happy-Go-Yoga might surprise you! If you're open to anything, put *Happy-Go-Yoga* in your bag right now and use it everywhere. We made it small, light, and portable for that reason.

So go—do some yoga your way, anywhere, anytime. Feel better more often. Devote yourself to you. Each day, you might be a little more happy-go-lucky with Happy-Go-Yoga in your life!

chapter two

Travel Buddies

Relief for your back, body, and mind during long flights and challenging commutes

Very rarely do I finish a flight or a train ride, emerge, and say, "OMG, I feel amazing!" Mass-transit travel is one of the hardest things on your body and soul.

For a national health blog, I interviewed a White House doctor, Connie Mariano, MD, who had been the presidential physician during three administrations (George H. W. Bush, Bill Clinton, and George W. Bush). She gave high marks to President Clinton for power napping, because, she told me, the more you sleep, the more you let your body restore itself. I couldn't agree more!

I say, use transit and flight time to give yourself that little health nap. On a train, close your eyes (but obviously don't miss your stop).

When you're *not* napping, make the most of your transit time with *Happy-Go-Yoga* Travel Buddies—poses that are good for the mind and body, from point A to point B.

In this chapter:

Eagle Perch ▪ **Eagle Twist** ▪ **Bird's Eye** ▪ **Bird of Prey**

Hang Time ▪ **Grounded in a Good Way** ▪ **Reach for the Moon**

Walk Your Puppies ▪ **Pray to the Seat Pocket** ▪ **Smooth Landing**

Eagle Perch

relieve ▪ strengthen ▪ focus ▪ empower ▪ relax

Stuck in a middle seat, your neck and shoulders are already tight, and you just started the flight. Two armrest hogs are making you feel worse. A few minutes start to feel like hours, and the dread is building for the journey ahead. Assume the perch of an eagle about to take flight and let your spirits soar (a little more).

Happy-Go-Yoga

1. Strap yourself in. Scoot your tailbone into the seat back so you can sit taller and be supported.

2. Don't arch your back to sit up, but lift the top of your head as if it could reach the ceiling of the plane.

3. Bend your arms at the elbows and raise your elbows to the height of your shoulders (stay within your space, please).

4. Choose one of the options below:

    Option A: Stack one elbow inside the other and connect the backs of your hands.

    Option B: Double wrap your arms and connect your palms.

    Option C: Press your arms together, elbows to palms.

5. In all options, feel the tops of your shoulders dropping away from your ears. Move just your elbows forward slightly toward the seat in front of you without changing the height of the arms.

6. Feel the stretch in your shoulders, upper arms, neck, and back.

7. Breathe easily and evenly. Count to ten slowly.

8. Switch sides (for option C, release and repeat).

Tip: Let your eagle circle in flight. Keep the pose (options A, B, or C) as you had it, but draw imaginary small, slow circles with your elbows.

About Eagle Perch

Based on Eagle Pose (Garudasana: *GAH-roo-DAH-suh-nuh*), Happy-Go-Yoga's Eagle Perch helps alleviate tight shoulders, stretches the upper back, and supports blood flow to help prevent muscle cramps and stiffness. With your arms in front of your eyes, you're forced to reevaluate your focus and concentration, which you'll need to resist the urge to elbow your rowmates. By the way, in yogic mythology, Garuda is the king of birds, eager to help humanity battle demons (aka inconsiderate fellow travelers).

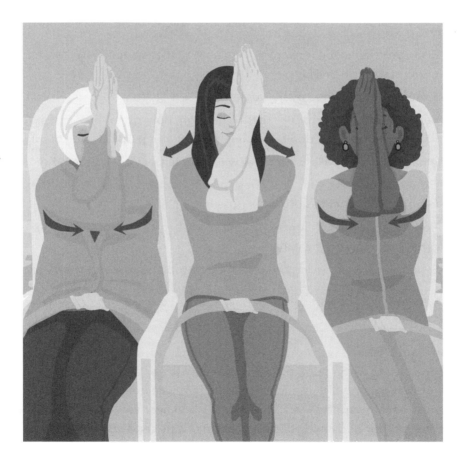

Eagle Twist

relieve ▪ de-stress ▪ relax

You've been staring at the seat pocket in front of you for quite some time now and studied the appropriate pictures in case of a water landing. Your lower back is tight and you start to wonder if the flight attendant would let you lie down in the aisle after beverage service ends. Here's a little twist on a tough yoga pose to melt the tight spots in your back.

Happy-Go-Yoga

1. Strap yourself in. Sit forward in your seat a little; sit up straight and comfortably (don't slump).

2. Cross your right knee over your left.

3. Put your left palm on your outer right thigh; hold on to the armrest with your right hand, but don't let your shoulder creep up toward your ear.

4. Inhale, and apply slight pressure with your left palm onto the outer thigh.

5. Exhale, and rotate your ribs, chest, and shoulders around to the right, keeping your chest as broad as possible.

6. Repeat steps 4 and 5 for two to four more breath rounds (inhale/exhale), always rotating on the exhale.

7. Switch sides by crossing the other leg on top and repeating the process.

EXTRA KARMA: As you twist, try to smile peacefully if you catch the gaze of someone across the aisle.

About Eagle Twist

Eagle Twist helps wring out the tightness in your lower back, a common place of discomfort on long flights and in general. The twist gently stretches the main back muscles that support the spine but are often overworked. Compressing the center of your body and your calf muscles helps send refreshing blood back into the muscles, organs, and spine when you untwist. Happy-Go-Yoga's Eagle Twist is a blend of the legs in Eagle Pose and Ardha Matsyendrasana (*ARD-uh MOTZ-ee-un-DRAH-suh-nuh*), a seated spinal twist, but it has an added health twist for travelers: It can also help encourage better digestion, which is always a plus when you're traveling and out of your regular routine.

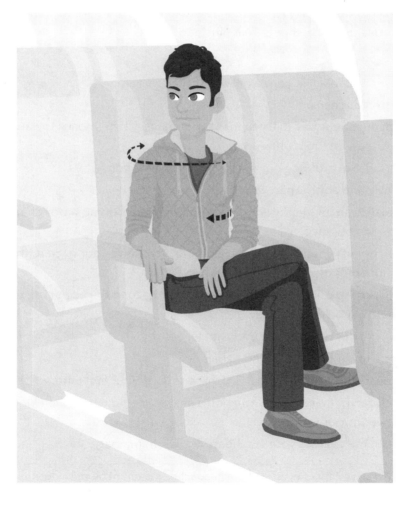

Bird's Eye

relieve ▪ focus ▪ relax ▪ refresh

Feeling headachy, you wonder if the airplane air is drying out your eyes. Between the track lighting and overhead reading light, your eyeballs hurt. Time to stretch your eyeballs (yes, eyeballs) instead of reaching for aspirin or a shot of vodka. Use this for a shot of relief instead.

Happy-Go-Yoga

1. Sit up and feel like you're growing taller.
2. Close your eyes.
3. Lift your shoulders to try to meet your ears, roll them back toward your seat, then let them relax away from your ears.
4. Let the skin around your eyes and your jaw soften.
5. Slowly and softly open your eyes.
6. Visualize an imaginary warm, indigo-blue line forming a box shape around your face.
7. Moving just your eyeballs and nothing else, send your gaze to the upper right corner of the box. Inhale and exhale.
8. Still moving only your eyeballs, shift your gaze to the upper left corner of the box. Inhale and exhale.
9. Then, lower right. Inhale and exhale.
10. Then, lower left. Inhale and exhale.
11. Repeat steps 7 through 10. Try three rounds your first time.
12. Reclose your eyes softly. Imagine a soft, soothing indigo-blue light in between your eyebrows.
13. Feel it melt across your forehead, like warm massage oil.

Note: If Bird's Eye causes eyestrain or a headache, you might be pushing your eyes too much—the movement of your eyeballs should be soft, like a gaze, not a hard stare.

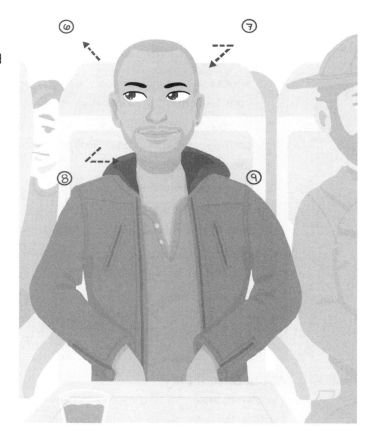

About Bird's Eye

Indigo blue is the color representing the wise energy point known as the "third eye" (Ajna Chakra: *ODJ-nuh CHUH-kruh*), related to focus, knowledge, and intuition. Moving the eyeballs on a course for all four corners of your imaginary box is a variation on Kundalini eye kriyas (*KREE-yuhs*), in which repetition of a certain movement or breath is meant to cleanse. The idea of a warm massage oil spreading across your forehead is inspired by shirodhara (Sanskrit for "head" and "flow"; *SHEER-oh-DARR-uh*), a traditional treatment that can be used to help a variety of eye diseases and promote relaxation. Consider Bird's Eye a way of relaxing, cleansing your eye discomfort, and clearing the clutter in your head for better focus and intuition.

Bird of Prey

de-stress ▪ focus ▪ empower ▪ brighten ▪ strengthen

Crumpled in your seat, you feel listless and zoned out, but not in a good way. You need to perk up and get some work done while you're in the air. Take a cue from powerful birds of prey, such as falcons and owls, and use special wings to posture yourself for productivity.

Happy-Go-Yoga

1. Scoot forward in your seat, leaving about three or four inches between your back and the seat back.

2. Wrap one arm behind your mid-back with the elbow bent so that your palm faces the seat back. Roll that shoulder slightly up and back toward the seat back.

3. If you feel comfortable, wrap your other arm behind in the same way. Grab opposite elbows.

4. Puff up your chest, but don't strain into a backbend.

5. Pretend that your collarbones are wings and they are reaching out to expand your wingspan on either side of your body.

6. Breathe deeply.

Note: Consider taking your Bird of Prey into other environments to feel a little more proactive and ready for the task ahead—say, when trapped at your desk on deadline.

About Bird of Prey

If you've ever seen a bird eyeing its prey, you'll notice concentration and poise. Raptors, for example, generally have well-developed senses and great vision, making them swift and effective in their tasks. Happy-Go-Yoga's Bird of Prey helps you take that shape and character as you lift up your body and strengthen your posture, based on a well-loved yoga arm position that opens up the front of the chest and shoulders (like a bird about to take off with purpose). By the way, did you know owls have a special feather structure that reduces turbulence, making for smoother flight? Let's hope you have a smooth flight, too.

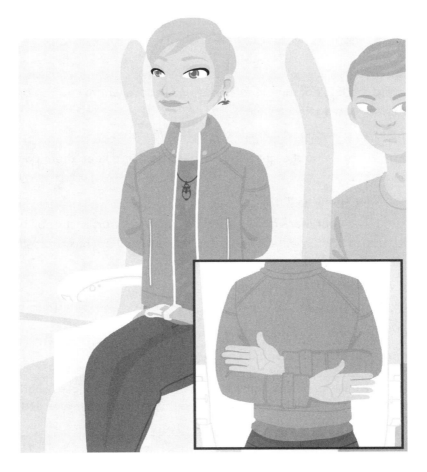

Hang Time

relieve ▪ **calm** ▪ **refresh** ▪ **strengthen**

You're craning your neck to see when the drink cart is coming down the aisle, and you think maybe a little cocktail would help release the crimp in your neck. Let the cart pass, take a breath, and head for the space at the back of the plane to release your neck instead. (You can do this waiting for the bus or in the train terminal, too. Just find a wall and a little space.)

Happy-Go-Yoga

1. Toward the back of the plane, find a small space where you can have your rear end against a wall.
2. Step away from the wall about ten to twelve inches.
3. Step your feet about eight to ten inches apart, and keep them parallel to one another.
4. Bend your knees a little bit.
5. As you lean your rear end against the wall for support and stability, fold your upper body over your legs, but lift your belly up into yourself a little to support your back.
6. Let your upper back feel softly rounded.
7. Let your head hang.
8. Hold your elbows with opposite hands.
9. Gently nod and shake your head to let some tension go.

Note: You might think it's odd to do this in public at first, but you'll feel so good, you really won't care who's watching. In truth, they're probably curious, envious, and thinking about copying you!

About Hang Time

Happy-Go-Yoga's Hang Time is a gentler version of a deep, calming pose, Standing Forward Fold (Uttanasana: *OOT-uh-NAH-suh-nuh*). Lifting your belly as you fold over your body helps strengthen your core (think fab abs). Bending your knees slightly gives your legs and rear end a little workout while the plane wall supports your balance. As you grab opposing elbows, your shoulders, upper arms, and back get a stretch from the gravity you create with your hang time here. Blood flows to the brain when you hang your head, quieting the mind and refreshing you from mind-numbing travel. As you jet across time zones, see if you can opt for some hang time instead of a Bloody Mary.

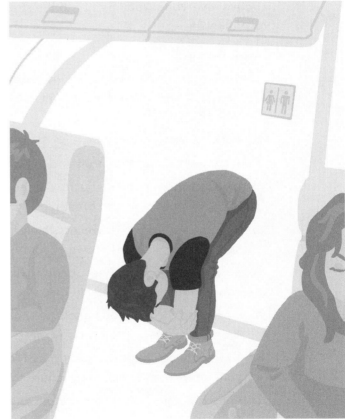

Grounded in a Good Way

strengthen • balance • focus

Your flight is grounded, literally. Weary, defeated, and impatient, you feel shrunken by airports, long lines, and travel stress—but you're not mentally grounded in a way that helps you cope, so you are primed to fly off the handle at everyone. You need both the strength and flexibility of a strong, graceful tree.

Happy-Go-Yoga

1. Stand next to your extended luggage handle, a wall, or a guardrail and hold it very lightly with your right hand. Don't lean on it or put a lot of weight on it.
2. Put your left hand on your hip.
3. Put your feet together, toes and heels touching or close together.
4. Deepen your breath in the area of the lower rib cage, expanding your ribs, like a balloon, with breath.
5. Imagine your breath traveling slowly from the earth, up your legs and spine, and toward the crown of your head. Keep breathing.
6. Slowly slide your left heel up the ankle toward your calf. (You can keep your toes on the ground if it helps you balance.)
7. Don't grip the luggage handle. Rely more on your standing foot and draw your navel into your body.
8. Keep connecting your standing foot to the earth and feel like the top of your head (not your chin) continues to lift.
9. Keep breathing fully in the middle of your body.
10. Switch sides.

Bonus: You can also try this without holding on to anything—just balance!

About Grounded in a Good Way

Trees, like this pose, are rooted and grounded so they can stay stable in the midst of swirling winds and rainy days. Use this active standing pose to keep your mind off negative things—like delays and crazy travelers—or do it without the luggage to stay stable while waiting in long lines anywhere. Grounded in a Good Way is Happy-Go-Yoga's take on the very popular Tree Pose (Vrksasana: *vrik-SHAH-suh-nuh*), which tones leg muscles and helps with stiffness in your legs and hips. It also gives you a sense of balance and poise as you breathe, grow tall, and focus on staying calm instead of obsessing about things that are out of your control.

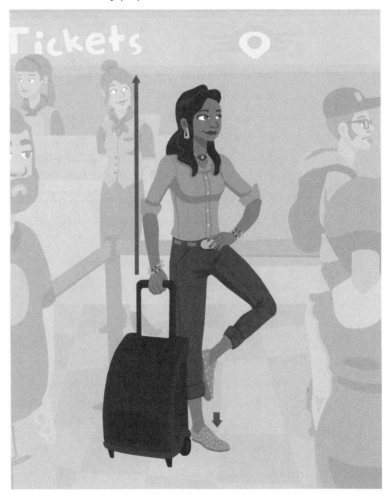

Reach for the Moon

relieve ▪ **strengthen** ▪ **brighten** ▪ **refresh**

You just missed out on getting a seat on the train, and you're standing. You're so tired that just sitting down would feel like a trip to the spa right about now. Time to stand your ground, give yourself a quick shot of energy, and reflect on the best parts of your day—rather than the worst—to arrive in peace.

Happy-Go-Yoga

1. Stand tall and inhale as you reach one arm above your head toward an overhead bar or handle. Let your other arm rest by your side.

2. As you reach for the bar, let the back of your shoulder drop toward your waist, and try to keep your arm straight, but not locked. (If you're a tall person, you might reach beyond the bar and press your inner arm or wrist into the bar, keeping your arm firm and stretched to its full length.)

3. Inhale, get taller, and exhale into a gentle side bend reaching your extended arm up and over your head while your other arm stays by your side.

4. As you make this crescent moon shape with your body, try not to collapse into your chest, but keep it open; feel your ribs lift off your hips for more breathing room.

5. Inhale and exhale at least five times. On each inhale, gaze up at the train ceiling in the direction of your upper arm and remember something good from the day—no matter how small. On each exhale gaze in the opposite direction over your other shoulder and toward the floor.

6. On the last exhale, come out of the side bend.

7. Be a little flexible in your grip to accommodate any unexpected movement by the train.

Tip: This pose is best done on an express train or longer section of a ride when there's not a lot of starting or stopping. You can also do this anytime you're standing for a long time—just pretend you have an overhead bar and reach up and over for the moon.

About Reach for the Moon

Anytime you feel sluggish, you can refresh yourself with Happy-Go-Yoga's version of a pose traditionally called Standing Half Moon. It strengthens the muscles along your spine and core and helps keep your back flexible in general as you make the shape of a crescent moon. The combination of neck and breathing movement is a Viniyoga therapy technique to break patterns of tense holding— here, we do it for your neck to alleviate neck and shoulder stiffness. The moon itself is calming and grounding. It also reflects the sun's light, which illuminates your unique wisdom and intuition. The crescent moon can also symbolize new beginnings and dreams that will become reality if you can let go of what brings you down.

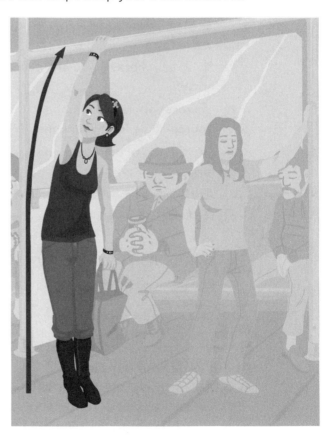

Walk Your Puppies

relieve ▪ strengthen ▪ refresh

All you want to do right now is kick off your shoes, but one glance at the subway floor…yeah, that's not going to happen. Wherever you are, you can give your tired puppies some TLC. Walk 'em a little so you're ready to trot to your next stop, which is hopefully home sweet home (or somewhere that will make you happy).

Happy-Go-Yoga

1. Sit up tall wherever you are (even if you're still checking your phone and email).
2. Uncross your legs and unbend them so they're at about a forty-five-degree angle from your knees as you sit.
3. Flex the top of one foot to bring your toes in the direction of your knee (up).
4. At the same time, press the entire bottom of the other foot on the floor.
5. Hold the positions from steps 3 and 4, and inhale and exhale deeply one time.
6. Switch sides, but don't speed up your breath or your walk.
7. Repeat steps 2 through 6 about a dozen times.

Bonus: For extra stretching and relief, during step 4, you could point the toe of the foot that's pressing into the floor, which will lift your heel and stretch the top of that foot.

About Walk Your Puppies

Based on yoga's popular Downward-Facing Dog (Adho Mukha Svanasana: *UDD-oh MOO-kuh schvah-NAH-suh-nuh*), which calms the brain and helps bring back lost energy, this Happy-Go-Yoga pose also can help relieve pain in your feet and heels. It creates strength and flexibility in your ankles and legs, too. According to Chinese traditional medicine, healing and well-being is supported when you take care of your feet! As you breathe and pedal your feet, you're basically "walking your (downward) dog." Your tired puppies will be less stiff and more energized. Isn't that what happens with dogs, too, when they get that long overdue stretch? Just remember to breathe while you walk, and wag your tail, always.

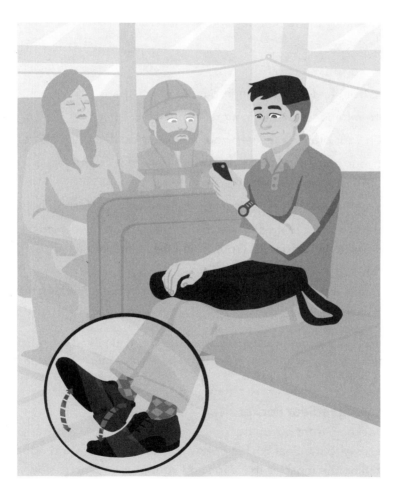

Pray to the Seat Pocket

relieve ▪ relax ▪ refresh ▪ balance

You thought there was only an hour left in your flight, but turns out it's only been an hour since you boarded. You're a bit deflated. You'll need some oxygen (that doesn't come from the air masks in case of an emergency) to refresh yourself for the remainder of the flight. You can do this on a long bus or train ride, too.

Happy-Go-Yoga

1. Place both feet on the floor about hip width apart.
2. Put your hands together in a prayer position.
3. Lift up your prayer and keep your elbows shoulder width apart.
4. Rest your elbows lightly on the seat in front of you, and let your prayer rest on the top of your head.
5. Gaze at the seat pocket in front of you and imagine feeling light as air.
6. Inhale as much breath as you can into the section of your ribs right underneath your armpits. (You should feel a little stretch if you get a lot of air in there.)
7. Gradually walk your elbows up the seat back after a few breaths, keeping the elbows level.

Tip: For extra breathing room and an extra stretch, you might bend your elbows more and set them on the top of the seat in front of you, resting your palms on the back of your neck.

About Pray to the Seat Pocket

The seat pocket in front of you becomes your peace altar in this Happy-Go-Yoga pose. Pray to the Seat Pocket opens up your shoulders and upper rib cage, stretching the muscles that surround your ribs, and increasing your ability to breathe deeply and relax. Yogis do this all the time in classes to get ready for a really hard upside down balance called Forearm Stand (Pincha Mayurasana: *PINCH-uh-MY-ur-AH-suh-nuh*), but, let's be honest, we really don't want to be upside down mid-flight, do we? This will do. Remember to let your elbows rest *lightly* on the seat in front of you. If you go a little too heavy and disturb the person in front of you, you'd better pray he or she is very understanding about your need for a little extra elbow room.

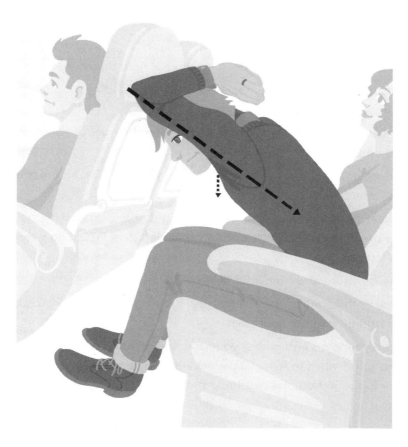

Smooth Landing

balance ▪ calm ▪ refresh

There's nothing like coming home, getting to your destination after a long journey, or feeling like you're safely back on the ground. If touchdown is a little bumpy, though, your nerves might get slightly shaken. Use this breathing technique to get calm and balanced, assuring a smooth landing, mentally.

Happy-Go-Yoga

1. As you taxi to the gate, close your eyes and sit up straight.
2. Bring your right hand toward your face.
3. Lightly close off your right nostril with your right thumb.
4. Through your left nostril, inhale smoothly (no gasping) and then exhale smoothly. Do this three times.
5. Lightly close off your left nostril with the fourth finger of your right hand and open your right nostril.
6. Repeat step 4, breathing through your right nostril. Three breaths…slow and smooth.
7. Repeat steps 3 and 4, closing off your right nostril again with the thumb and breathing deeply three times on the left side. (You'll do it twice on the left side.)
8. Release your hand from your face.
9. Place both palms on your thighs and breathe through both nostrils for a few breaths without counting.
10. Open your eyes and gather your belongings with composure, and try to send good vibes to fellow travelers who are less composed as they grab their luggage from the overhead bin.

Note: You can do this breathing exercise anywhere you need a balanced feeling—say, when barely making it to a doctor's appointment, only to sit in the waiting room for a few minutes. Do Smooth Landing to reduce your blood pressure slightly before the nurse takes it!

About Smooth Landing

Learning how to control your breathing is a staple in yoga. Happy-Go-Yoga's Smooth Landing is an adaptation of Alternate Nostril Breath (Nadi Shodhana: *nah-dee SHO-dunn-uh*), a particular breath technique used to create a balance between the dueling parts of the nervous system—one that kicks you into gear when you need to take action, and the other, which helps you rest and restore. Breathing through your right nostril is energizing, while breathing on the left side is more calming, which is why, in this version, we start and end on the left side. Smooth Landing helps stabilize a rattled mind and synchronize our systems, which, for most of us, is a little wonky during travel, especially after a not-so-smooth touchdown.

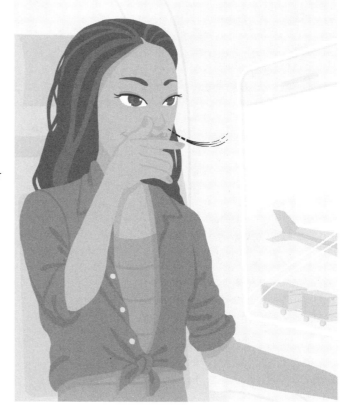

chapter three

Career Counselors

On-the-job strategies for stress relief, focus,
confidence, and productivity

You work hard for the money! Sometimes, though, work is a little harder than you'd like. *Sigh.* You can't control gossiping coworkers or getting a massive assignment at the last minute; however, you can manage your own cubicle aches and work stress without taking up a lot of time in your work schedule.

Studies show that a little mindful movement throughout the day can make a big difference in both mental and physical health. There's also research from Harvard claiming that certain "power poses" can help you build confidence for that job interview or big presentation. Who knew? Well, the yogis did, long ago…

If you need to, schedule a Happy-Go-Yoga minute or two on your calendar, and make an appointment for a well-deserved and critical health break. (Yes, it's okay if your smartphone alarm reminds you to do yoga. Just choose a soothing ringtone like a harp or something, please.)

When you feel ready to work again, you'll be more productive. You'll also be easier to work *with*…which is always a good career move.

In this chapter:

Wrist Wrestling · **Confidence Booster** · **Twist, Don't Shout** · **Total Brain Power** · **Stand Your Ground** · **Let It Roll** · **Spine Align** · **Forgive the Frenemy** · **Counter Pose** · **Office Warrior**

Wrist Wrestling

relieve • refresh

It's time for computer detox. No doubt you've been typing like a maniac, trying to finish your project, but an endless stream of emails keeps interrupting you. Give your hands and wrists a little boost so they can keep going. Challenge them to a wrist-wrestling match right at your desk.

Happy-Go-Yoga

1. Look away from your screen (at something calm, like a plant).
2. Gently reach both arms in front of you and keep your elbows slightly bent.
3. Interlace your fingers and press your palms together steadily, without gripping hard.
4. Draw a slow figure eight shape with your knuckles in one direction, moving from your wrists.
5. Breathe slowly, too.
6. Switch directions (this might be harder than you think).
7. Try it for twenty or thirty seconds—the wrestling match doesn't have to last long to be a good one!

About Wrist Wrestling

Wrists are pretty small joints compared to the rest of the body, but we ask them to do a lot in our device-obsessed world: typing, texting, emailing, gaming, and more. If they're in the same position for long periods of time as you type at the keyboard, you're not letting your wrists enjoy their full range of motion. They'll get stiff and lazy, which is a recipe for pain. Yogis don't have a Sanskrit name for this one, but they know how to take care of the wrists. We do this all the time in class after balancing on our hands and after many Downward-Facing Dogs. Wrist Wrestling is a simple motion, but by giving your wrists a little twist and flow, you bring blood flow back to your hands, allowing you to wrestle your project with renewed spirit and vigor flowing from your fingertips.

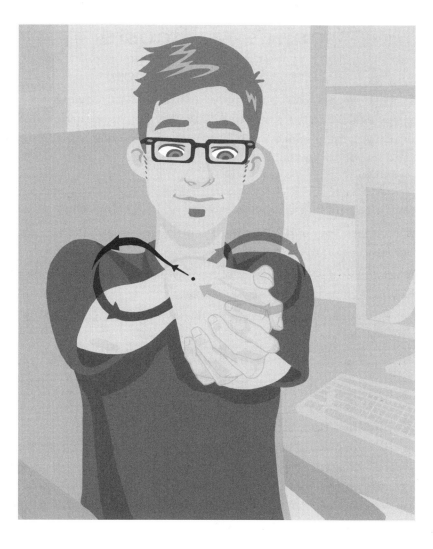

Confidence Booster

de-stress ▪ **inspire** ▪ **focus** ▪ **empower**

The boss is in the room, you're hoping for a raise, and your coworker is throwing you a fake grin that's making you uneasy. You need to look and sound like you're on your game. Take two minutes—just two minutes—go somewhere private, and let your *body* tell your *mind*, "You got this."

Happy-Go-Yoga

1. Stand with your feet parallel to each other. They can be slightly apart.
2. As you reach your arms downward, feel your chest and the very top of your head lifting to the ceiling.
3. Try not to bend your back a lot or throw your chin to the sky; instead, feel like you're growing taller—soaring, maybe!
4. Breathe deeply. Your exhale can be a little longer than your inhale to help calm your nerves.
5. Do this for just two minutes to feel a real confidence boost.

Tip: Not to be done in the actual meeting room. Go somewhere private.

About Confidence Booster

Standing tall is the basis of yoga's Mountain Pose (Tadasana: *tuh-DAHS-uh-nuh*). Harvard researchers have actually put their stamp of approval on these types of poses, which mimic the body shapes of winning athletes: chest high, head high with an upward motion in their bodies; in a word, victorious! When you put your body in a shape that's victorious, you emit more testosterone, the dominance hormone, and less cortisol, the stress hormone. Confidence Booster puts you in this shape and empowers you to pay better attention, remember more clearly, perform well, and sense your surroundings. Physically, by bearing weight evenly in the feet, the rest of your body can be lighter, and your mind can soar with agility and a winning attitude.

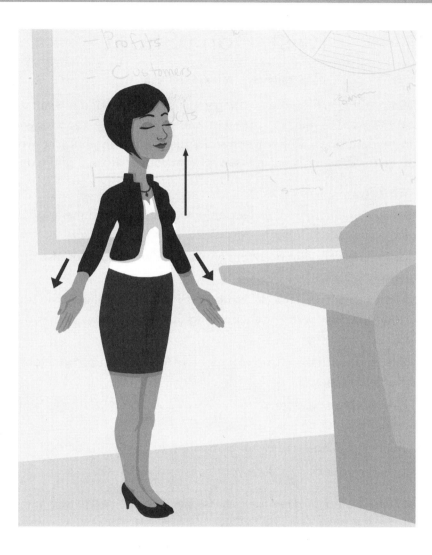

Twist, Don't Shout

relieve ▪ relax ▪ refresh

Knots in your stomach from the meeting you just left? You kind of want to shout out "@!$%#&" to release frustration. This would not be good for your job review. Instead, sit down for a twist on stress relief and wring out your worries. Let go of the toxic feeling that'll just eat away at you for the rest of the day.

Happy-Go-Yoga

1. Sit in a chair that rotates, but scoot forward a bit toward the edge of the seat.

2. Face the desk and put both feet on the floor with your toes also facing the desk.

3. Put your left palm on the desk and press your right palm on the seat next to your right rear, with fingers pointing outward and away from your body.

4. Inhale, and reach the crown of your head to the ceiling so you feel your spine getting longer.

5. Exhale, and twist your torso to the right as you draw your belly button deeper into your center.

6. Repeat steps 4 and 5 a few times, twisting deeper with each exhale.

7. Reposition your body to face your desk and switch sides.

Tip: Twist, Don't Shout should feel like a release, not an assignment to twist as much as possible. No one's measuring your progress here, so just let go and twist until you release the need to shout, "@!$%#&".

About Twist, Don't Shout

Happy-Go-Yoga's Twist, Don't Shout is the upright version of a reclined twist called Stomach-Revolving Spinal Twist (Jathara Parivartanasana: *juh-TAR-uh par-EE-var-tuh-NAH-suh-nuh*). Twists are detoxifying and sometimes can help get rid of that sinking feeling in your gut. They also have the ability to restore or keep suppleness in your lower-back muscles, which get stiff and sore from sitting in those long meetings. Twisting is a basic part of any yogi's life, meant to calm anxiety and relieve sluggishness by bringing a "wring-out-and-release" action to your body's digestion and nourishment organs. When stuff keeps moving in this area, you regularly purge the toxins that don't support your vitality while you circulate the energy and fuel that does. It's true, sometimes shouting just feels good, but twisting might be a better way to avoid being called to Human Resources.

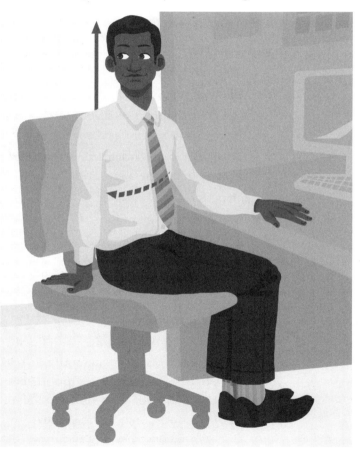

Total Brain Power

focus ▪ balance ▪ empower

You can't quite put your finger on it, but you feel like a part of your brain isn't working, and you really have to concentrate to get the job done on time. It'll only take a minute to make a positive hand gesture to clear your mind and spark mental power throughout all parts of your brain.

Happy-Go-Yoga

1. Sit comfortably.
2. Join your hands at your fingertips and thumbs.
3. Bring this shape toward your forehead and touch your thumbs to the space between your eyebrows, but just a little higher.
4. Close your eyes, and imagine a midnight-blue sky that's clear, with no clouds but maybe a few bright stars.
5. Inhale for a count of four.
6. Exhale for a count of four.
7. Repeat steps 4 and 5 ten times.

Tip: Your shoulders might start to drift up and create tension in your neck. Use your back muscles to move them down so you don't drain the power-up process.

About Total Brain Power

Hakini is the god of the forehead, and the inspiration for Happy-Go-Yoga's Total Brain Power. This is Hakini mudra (*HAH-kee-nee MOOD-ruh*). Mudras are yoga of the hands, and this one supports mental clarity. By putting all your fingers and your thumbs together, you balance all the natural elements and energies of the body, uniting the creative and analytical sides of the brain. When signals are crisscrossing randomly, Total Brain Power can help promote cooperation instead so everything works together as a unit. This mudra is also said to improve breathing. You'll need that oxygen to feed your brain for maximum productivity. Totally.

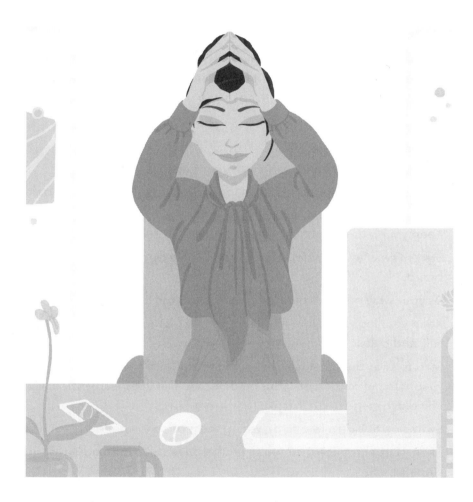

Stand Your Ground

empower ▪ strengthen ▪ balance

There's a lot of change happening at work, all at once! You're feeling a little off balance, unstable, and worried about many things. It's time to get grounded so you have a foundation to be flexible, no matter what happens. Don't worry. It's going to be okay.

Happy-Go-Yoga

1. Take your shoes off, and stand with your feet together.
2. Lift your toes off the ground, then lower them to feel the ground beneath you.
3. Keep your legs straight, and imagine that your ankles are hinges.
4. Start to sway to one side, keeping your whole body firm as if it were a board.
5. As your sway gets to its farthest point, your other foot will peel off the floor.
6. Keep your legs firm, your lifted foot flat, as if it were standing on the floor still, and balance momentarily.
7. Start to sway the other way, keeping the legs firm and transferring the weight to the other foot. (Your other foot will lift in similar fashion as the first did in step 5.)
8. Sway side to side a few times, taking the motion to your edge each time.
9. Then, start to reduce the motion until you are still and standing—as in steps 1 and 2.
10. Picture yourself firmly grounded in your own situation.

Tip: Try not to use your hips, lift your legs, or bend your knees to peel your foot off the ground when you sway. It should happen naturally. Focus more on balancing when it does happen. It's like life—sometimes you have to balance things when they decide to happen. You can't control them!

About Stand Your Ground

When you're rooted firmly at the base, you can handle anything that blows your way. Happy-Go-Yoga's Stand Your Ground is a blend of the traditional foot lock called Pada Bandha (*PUDD-uh BUN-dah*) and a balance technique to connect your entire foot base to the earth for maximum stability and steadiness in the midst of really challenging yoga poses. Just doing Stand Your Ground helps strengthen your spine and core to improve posture. As you sway, you'll strengthen your legs, core, and ankles, too. When you come back to stillness, you'll be more aware of the difference between being off balance and being stable, which will help you be more aware of how to come back into balance when things knock you off your feet a little. One of my favorite inspirational quotes is an old Japanese proverb: "The bamboo that bends is stronger than the oak that resists." Root deeply, but be flexible!

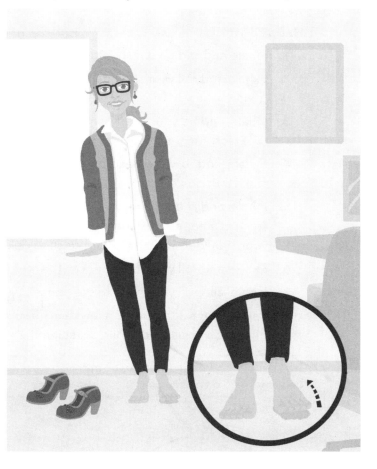

Let It Roll

relieve ▪ brighten ▪ relax

You just noticed that the knots in your neck are the size of your ears. (Maybe this is an exaggeration, okay, but it sure feels tight up there.) You're probably not letting enough roll off your shoulders, and those knots are blocking your creative energy. Let it roll and release the weight of the world so you can express yourself.

Happy-Go-Yoga

1. Inhale and shrug your shoulders to the ears.
2. Exhale and roll your shoulders back, letting them fall away from the ears gently.
3. Inhale, and tip your head gently to the right, bringing your right ear a little closer to your shoulder without lifting the shoulder to it.
4. Exhale, and roll your head so your chin gets a little tucked toward your chest (but don't strain).
5. Inhale, and keep rolling your head in the same direction, to the left, so it lands in a tipped position to the left, and your left ear is a little closer to your shoulder without lifting your shoulder to meet your ear.
6. Exhale and roll your head back to the middle. Tuck your chin gently.
7. Inhale, and roll your head to the right.
8. Repeat steps 3 through 7 a few times. You should start to notice the difference in just a few rolls, so let it roll.

Tip: If you are particularly tense, you may need to repeat steps 1 and 2 a few times before moving on to step 3.

About Let It Roll

When something unexpected happens, the body's natural nervous-system response is to tense up and/or hunch over to protect and get ready to defend. If you keep doing this, though, your muscles will start to think that fear is the new normal and will stay stiff and knotted. Keep it rolling, and your neck muscles soften. Over time, they'll just be more adaptable and flexible. Let It Roll, Happy-Go-Yoga style, to relieve neck tightness right away. Do it regularly to retrain your muscles and your mind to manage the unexpected stuff a little more easily. By the way, giving your neck space also helps creativity flow, because it unblocks the subtle energy of the Vishuddha Chakra (*vish-YOO-duh CHUH-kruh*), which rules one's ability to express, be creative, and communicate confidently.

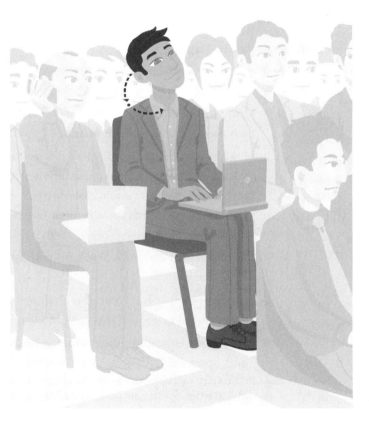

Spine Align

relieve • balance • refresh

You're losing steam at your computer. Possible explanations for this:
1) your body is working too hard while sitting, or 2) just sitting there for too long is draining the specific type of health energy needed for important things on the job. Here's one way that yogis restore that energy. You need a bath towel, a thick scarf, or a thin blanket for this one.

Happy-Go-Yoga

1. First, get up from your desk and stretch (any stretch, I'm begging you).

2. Take a deep breath in, hold it at the top of your breath for a moment, then open your mouth and release a big sigh to let go of tension (or whatever is causing you tension).

3. Prep the roll: Roll up your towel/scarf/blanket as shown in the illustration. (Don't rush this part: take the time to make it smooth and flat before you roll it up. You don't want a bumpy roll—bad for the back.) Try to let the roll be about as long as the distance between your seat and the base of your neck.

4. Align the roll vertically along your spine, between your back and your chair back.

5. Scoot your rear back into the chair to secure the base of the roll where it touches the corner of the seat and the seat back.

6. Lean back onto the roll and feel your shoulders and chest stretch wider and open up.

Tip: I love this one for the airplane seats, too, though they really don't give you blankets anymore. You'll have to pack a thick scarf in your carry-on.

About Spine Align

Happy-Go-Yoga's Spine Align is based on a technique in the Restorative yoga practice, which helps your body find its natural comfort zone and restore energy. The roll itself can help align your spine to relieve neck, shoulder, and back tightness by readjusting your body so it's not working so hard just to sit. All of this frees up energy for something better. Working long, consecutive hours at the computer robs your mind of energy and is one of the top zappers of *prana vayu* (*PRAH-nuh V'EYE-yoo*). Considered the most important movement energy, a balanced *prana vayu* supports your vision, hearing, creative thinking, reasoning, and enthusiasm. We need all of that to do a good job! I think that's worth keeping a scarf, towel, or blanket handy at work, don't you?

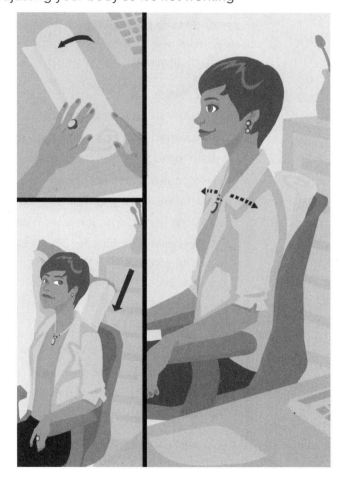

Forgive the Frenemy

de-stress ▪ **love** ▪ **connect**

Oh, there's that coworker who pretends to be your friend, but you know she's out to get you. (Okay, do you really know that? Really?) Maybe it's time to release and make peace within *you*. The power is in your hands to shift your energies from negative to positive and release internal toxicity—the bigger enemy to your health.

Happy-Go-Yoga

1. Sit at your desk, feet on the floor.
2. Sit up confidently and close your eyes.
3. Inhale through your nose; exhale and sigh out through your mouth.
4. Close your mouth and breathe through your nose.
5. With the backs of your hands on your knees, palms facing up, make fists with your hands, with the thumb crossing over the rest of the knuckles.
6. Release your fists, lift your hands off your knees, and bring your hands together along the pinkies, and make a bowl shape by cupping your hands.
7. Inhale, make the fists.
8. Exhale, make the bowl.
9. Inhale, make the fists and think, "Let…"
10. Exhale, make the bowl and think, "…go."
11. Repeat steps 7 and 8 a few more times, as needed to let negative feelings pass, or to feel a little forgiveness.

Tip: If your frenemy on the job has really been bugging you for a while, you might need to do this regularly, rather than just after a "situation." Think of it as giving yourself a bigger dose of the pose to get rid of the issue, then maintaining your health with regular treatment.

Extra Karma: Ask the Frenemy to lunch. I know, I know. Just try it?

About Forgive the Frenemy

Your hands are expressions of the heart, so use them to make ancient, powerful gestures that can shift your energy. With your fists in Forgive the Frenemy, you create Mushti mudra (*MOOSH-ti MOOD-ruh*). When you release your fists, you release pent-up emotions. The bowl with your hands is Pushpaputa mudra (*PUSH-puh-PUT-uh MOOD-ruh*), which means "handful of flowers" and is a symbol of receiving and offering peace. When you bite your tongue at work (and let's be honest, we've all been there), over time you hike your stress levels chronically and weaken your immune system. In other words, you hold it all in, and you're pretty much a sitting duck waiting to get every bad cold that goes around the office. Let the little stuff go quietly, then choose appropriate moments to stand your ground instead (refer to Happy-Go-Yoga's Stand Your Ground on page 40).

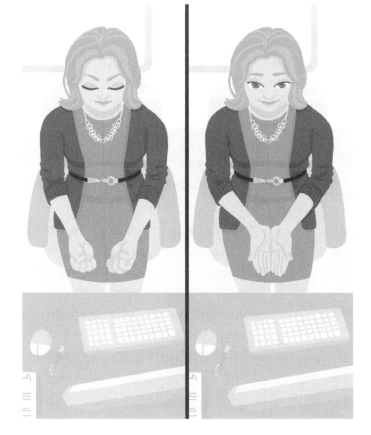

Counter Pose

relieve · balance · relax · calm

Ever the dedicated worker bee, you've lost track of how long you've been plugging away. Your hips and lower back are telling you it's time to take a break. In yoga, counterposes help even out the body after holding a certain shape. In real life, we need a counterpose for sitting at our desks for too long.

Happy-Go-Yoga

1. Stand, face your desk, and clear space right in front of you.

2. Stabilize yourself with your hands on the desk underneath your shoulders.

3. Lift your right leg and let your outer shin and calf rest on the desk. (Your knee should be on the desk, too, a little wider than the width of your shoulder. Move your right hand aside, but keep it on the desk.)

4. Flex your right foot, like you're moving your toes closer to your shin, and firm your foot, as if you're chopping the outer edge of your foot into the desk.

5. Lean a little (but not a lot) on your left hand.

6. Take the heel of your right palm close to the crease of your hip—on your thigh with your fingers pointing slightly outward toward your outer thigh.

7. Press down gently to rotate your thigh out and down toward the desk. (Do your best; this is challenging.) Try not to lean too much to one side or the other; keep your hips even to support your lower back.

8. If you're okay with step 7, keep everything the way it is and then lean forward toward your computer screen; hinge at your hips, evenly, with a flat back, to go deeper. Walk your fingertips forward on the desk to support you.

9. Breathe.

10. Repeat steps 3 through 9 for the left side.

Tip: This is a big release for the hips and lower back, but one of the most rewarding. Take it slow, do a little at a time, and don't force anything. Knee injuries? Be especially careful. Above all else, don't hold your breath—we're trying to release, and it helps to keep breathing.

About Counter Pose

Happy-Go-Yoga's Counter Pose is based on One-Legged King Pigeon (Eka Pada Rajakapotasana: *ECK-uh POD-uh ROJ-uh KUP-oh-TAHS-uh-nuh*). It's not as hard as it sounds! Counter Pose lengthens the psoas muscle of your hip flexor, which gets chronically shorter and shorter when we sit and sit. Counter Pose also helps keep your hip joint mobile to counteract the tightness that builds up from remaining seated. Folding forward over your leg and desk calms your mind, as do similar shapes in yoga. (As you fold forward, try not to spill anything on the important papers covering your desk. If that happens, refer to page 42 and try Let It Roll.)

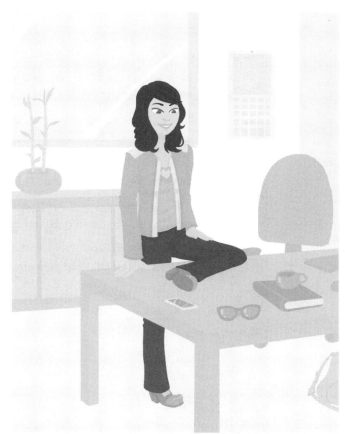

Office Warrior

empower ▪ **focus** ▪ **strengthen** ▪ **inspire**

"Is it Friday yet?" Oh right. It's only Tuesday. You could use a shot of steadiness to calm your nerves, plus a boost of power to stay motivated for everything you still have left on your to-do list. You're tempted to reach for an energy drink, but instead, draw upon the spirit of a fierce warrior to fuel your own personal power.

Happy-Go-Yoga

1. Find a chair with four solid legs (no wheels) in a spot where there's enough room behind you to stretch out your leg.

2. Stand, facing the back of the chair, and hold the top of the seat back with your hands, fingers over the top of the seat back.

3. Walk backward but don't let go of the chair. Put your feet together to touch, toes facing the back of the chair.

4. Think of a magnet keeping your inner thighs connected, then stretch one leg back into the air; keep it as straight as you can.

5. Reach more through your heel and keep your pinkie toe facing the floor (to keep the front of that hip pointing downward rather than opening up like a book).

6. Feel the floor evenly underneath you, and lean less on the chair.

7. Without sucking in your breath, feel like you are absorbing your belly button into yourself to firm your midsection, and keep breathing.

8. Repeat steps 4 through 7 with the other leg.

Bonus: Need more power and a bigger challenge? Take Office Warrior to the next level. Go back to step 3 and walk back farther to make an L shape with your body; your face and torso will face the floor, and your arms will be fully extended in a ninety-degree angle to the chair. Repeat steps 4 through 8.

About Office Warrior

Office Warrior is based on the challenging strength and focus-building Warrior III Pose (Virabhadrasana III: *VEER-uh-buh-DRAHS-uh-nuh*). This warrior pose brings together important yogic energy centers that benefit our own skills and abilities—it helps us feel more secure, builds our stamina so we can take risks, and supports strong self-esteem while connecting us with our own fearless will to face challenges. Physically, Office Warrior strengthens your core, back, arm, and leg muscles, while building balance and invigorating your entire body. It's a tough one, so it also forces you to concentrate in the moment. Have this moment. Then move on with your week. You can do it.

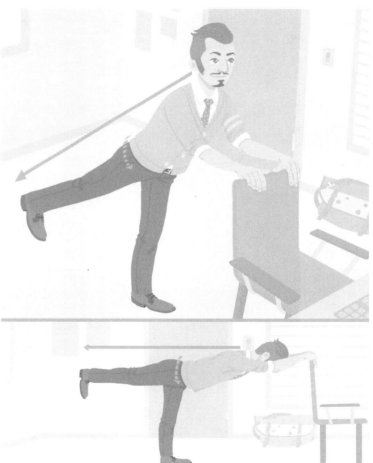

chapter four

Road Rage Relief

Stretches and tension tamers for intense traffic and long road trips

Road rage is kind of a retro term. It stuck with us after a slew of Los Angeles media reports in the '80s, but today, we use the term to describe all those special, stress-related behaviors that only seem to show up when you get in a car and drive. They get extra special when you're a daily commuter.

You know those ridiculous drivers who cross three lanes to cut you off and slam on the brakes, right? They're raging (yeah, just a little). Don't be that driver, and don't let that driver make *you* rage. Instead, keep your eyes on the road and use these Happy-Go-Yoga poses to feel more calm, comfortable, and collected each time you get behind the wheel for short drives or long road trips.

Think of them as your mind-body GPS system, keeping you safe and sane behind the wheel while guiding you to your destination of a healthier self.

The poses in this chapter have an added description, *HGY Travel Advisory*, so you can know when it's best to do them. Now you can be a yogi and a responsible driver at the same time.

In this chapter:

Car Kali ▪ **Nimble Warrior** ▪ **Road Hips** ▪ **Rearview Mirror**
Unlock Gridlock ▪ **Road Warrior I** ▪ **Road Warrior II** ▪ **Get Toe'd**
Parking Karma ▪ **Hey DJ**

Car Kali

empower ▪ **refresh** ▪ **inspire**

Time is ticking and you're late to your destination. Rather than drive like a crazy person, dodging cars and breaking laws, get a little crazy like Kali, the goddess of empowerment and transformation, for a more peaceful state of mind. She's known to clear the bad to make way for the good.

Happy-Go-Yoga

HGY Travel Advisory: Do this pose at a stoplight or while stopped in traffic.

1. Press your foot firmly on the brake or engage the emergency brake (this is important).
2. Cross your arms and hold on to the wheel.
3. Inhale a big, powerful breath into your body. Fill yourself up.
4. Stick your tongue out, exhale quickly, and make an ugly face and a fierce, monster-like noise when you let your breath out.
5. Right away, check back with the traffic in front of you to make sure you don't add to the gridlock.

Extra Karma: If you're still going nowhere after step 5, look out the window at another person stuck in gridlock and smile. Kids are great for this.

Note: Car Kali might seem a bit crazy, but do it once, and I'll bet you feel a big release!

About Car Kali

Happy-Go-Yoga's Car Kali (KAH-lee) liberates you from soul-draining frustration on the road. The goddess Kali is known to annihilate evil, which is not always a pretty sight. In fact, she's sometimes straight-up scary. Making a monstrous noise and ugly face stretches out your face muscles and skin, then releases you into a calmer place. The big noise will help you release feelings festering within. You have to be willing to go there with Car Kali, to make some real noise and get fierce in your expression. Transformation doesn't happen if your Car Kali sounds like a kitten purr.

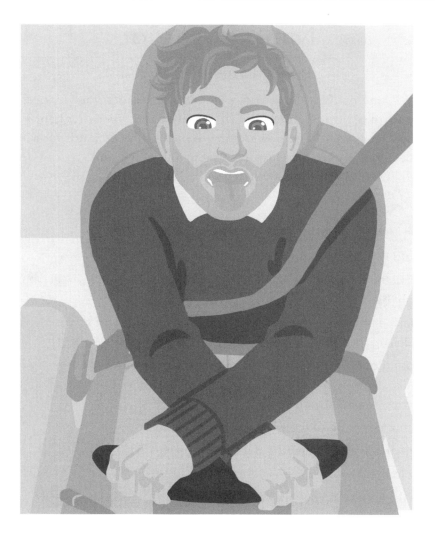

Nimble Warrior

relieve • de-stress • strengthen

Dodging in and out of traffic with the other road warriors, you've done your fair share of gripping the steering wheel—to the point your hands are cramping. Guess what? The power is in the palms of your hands for a little more peace rather than pressure. Be nimble and quick, and you can do this safely while you're waiting at the light.

Happy-Go-Yoga

HGY Travel Advisory: Best done when the car is stopped.

1. Hold the steering wheel with both hands.
2. Hold the wheel with the left hand while you release the wheel with your right hand.
3. Make a tight fist with your right hand and turn your fist so your wrist faces up.
4. Spring open your fist with the palm up. Keeping your wrist facing up, make another fist, and spring open. Make another first, and spring open (so, three times).
5. Then, take hold of the wheel with both hands.
6. Breathe in slowly. Breathe out slowly.
7. Hold the wheel with your right hand.
8. Make a fist with your left hand.
9. Repeat steps 3-6 with the left hand, then hold the wheel again with both hands as in step 5.
10. Breathe in. Breathe out.
11. Repeat as hand cramps occur.

Tip: Don't do this while switching lanes, trying to pick up your kids from school, or hunting down a parking space at the mall. That's not nimble. That's just nuts.

About Nimble Warrior

Happy-Go-Yoga's Nimble Warrior is inspired by a hand-flipping motion, commonly done when moving between two poses in the Warrior series: Warrior II and Peaceful Warrior, transitioning between ferocity and peace. By making a tight fist and then releasing it quickly, you're enhancing the release of blood flow to the muscles, joints, and tissues of the hands and wrists, which have been frozen in your grip of the wheel. Your arm muscles get in on the action as you flip the palm and make the grip, so there's a little strengthening in there for your biceps and triceps, too, in case traffic prevents you from getting to the gym (or yoga class) that day.

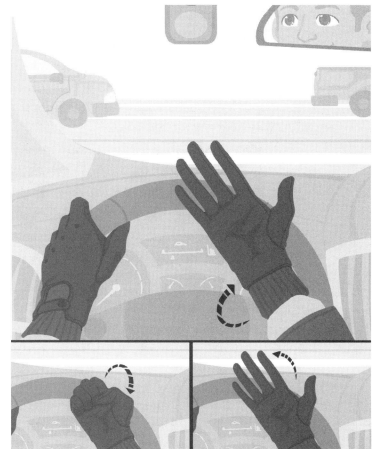

Road Hips

relieve ▪ strengthen

You've been behind the wheel for quite some time. You need a bathroom break and a stretch that'll help keep you perky for the rest of the road trip. Pull over at a rest stop or scenic viewpoint to relieve stiff hips and knees—and give your legs some energy for another stretch of road.

Happy-Go-Yoga

HGY Travel Advisory: Do this pose at a rest stop, scenic pullout, or similar place.

1. Stand still and tall (take advantage of the scenery).
2. Cross your right foot behind the left foot; try to have the full surface of both feet touch the ground. (Your right pinkie toe will probably be near the heel of your left foot.)
3. Inhale and reach your arms toward the sky.
4. Exhale, put your hands on your hips, and fold over toward both feet without bouncing, pushing down, or straining to touch your toes.
5. Keep both legs straight (or bend your knees slightly if you're tight in your back or hamstrings); keep both feet planted evenly as they stay crossed.
6. Stand back up, switch sides, and try to keep breathing smoothly.

Bonus: If your balance seems okay, let your head hang when you're folded over to get a good release for your neck, too.

Bonus: If you can, let go of your hips and reach toward an imaginary ten o'clock on the ground when your right foot is behind; two o'clock when your left foot is behind. Don't force it! Maybe your fingers touch the ground, maybe they don't—it doesn't matter! Your hips will still thank you!

About Road Hips

Road trips make you feel free to roam wherever your wheels can take you, but sitting behind the wheel for that long can trap your hips in a position that aggravates your lower body. Happy-Go-Yoga's Road Hips combines a forward bend that releases your lower back with a leg crossing to restore some suppleness in the iliotibial (IT) band, a band of tissues that runs from the top of the hips down the outside of the thigh. Tightness in the hips can travel around the lower back and down to the knee, common places of stiffness during long road trips. A few quick Happy-Go-Yoga Road Hips sprinkled throughout your trip, and you're good to go the distance.

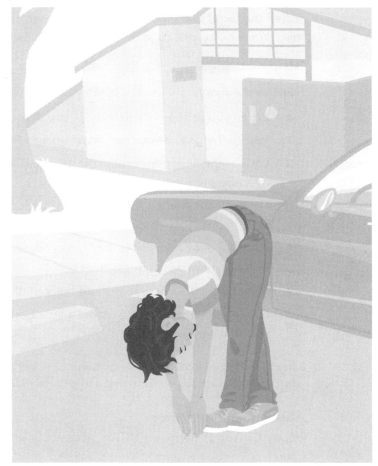

Rearview Mirror

relax ▪ de-stress ▪ calm ▪ brighten

Today has just not been a pretty day, and unfortunately, it's written all over your face. Examine your expression in the car's rearview mirror for a reality check. Soften the facial expression you see in the mirror to send a signal to yourself to relax. You'll be surprised at how quickly this one works.

Happy-Go-Yoga

HGY Travel Advisory: Best done when you are stopped at a light, firmly braking.

1. When you're at a complete stop, check yourself out in the mirror.
2. Ignore things like your hair, makeup, etc. Focus on your facial expression.
3. Look at the space between your brows. Is it furrowed? Lift your inner eyebrows to remove the wrinkles.
4. Look at your jaw. Is it clenched? Force a loose grin to get rid of the jaw lock.
5. Are your eyes angry? Think of how you would look at a person you love and put more of that into your gaze.
6. Notice how your face looks and feels a little nicer this way.
7. Give yourself permission to feel a little better right then and there and stay that way longer.

Note: Use Rearview Mirror wisely, as there is a risk of becoming too obsessed with how you look. Too much self-criticism and a huge ego are neither pretty nor relaxing!

About Rearview Mirror

Happy-Go-Yoga's Rearview Mirror gives you a way to let your body tell your mind to calm down quickly. Your body and your mind have a reciprocal relationship. When your body is healthier, your mind works better. When your mind is balanced between activity and rest, your body functions work better—digestion, sleep, and so on. You know the saying "seeing is believing"? You might not believe you're cranky, pissed, or stressed, but your face might say it for you. One look in the rearview mirror of your car will tell you all you need to know. You can tell your body—with your face—to leave the bummer day behind you and never look back.

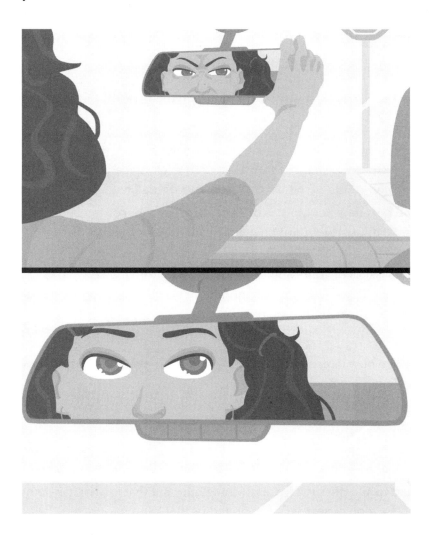

Unlock Gridlock

focus • calm • relieve • balance

Gridlock is in full swing, and your right leg is doing a dance: Accelerator. Brake. Accelerator. Brake. Brake lights and horns all around have made your eyes weary and overstimulated. Rebalance your seat and your sight to unlock some ease in the moment.

Happy-Go-Yoga

HGY Travel Advisory: Start when your foot is on the brake at a stop.

Your Seat

1. As you sit in the driver's seat, punching the pedals, notice that your right side is probably farther forward than the left, since you're actively using that entire side of the body in stop-and-go traffic.

2. The next time your foot is on the brake, use the resistance of the brake pedal to push your right hip backward, toward the seat back, and even it out with your left hip.

3. If the backs of your shoulders are far away from the seat back, adjust the seat forward so you're sitting more upright, stacking your shoulders directly above your even hips.

Your Sight

4. Notice how intensely you're glaring at the brake lights in front of you while people honk around you.

5. Start to reduce the intensity of your stare as it jumps from one thing to another.

6. Feel your gaze soften, and imagine your eyelids—and the skin around your eyes—softening as well, but keep your eyes open and alert.

7. Start to see the situation as a whole moment that is what it is, rather than a collection of several irritating things that keep happening.

Tip: If you only go as far as doing the first part of Gridlock—Your Seat—that's plenty! The concept of Your Sight will take a little more practice, as it is a more subtle practice of worrying less about the little things and remembering the big picture: that each breath is a blessing.

About Unlock Gridlock

Happy-Go-Yoga's Unlock Gridlock helps you change the way you sit and see so your body and eyes get relief from intense stop-and-go. As you bring your right hip back to match your left, then your torso over your hips, you line everything up so your spine and back muscles work together, rather than against you. Unlock Gridlock borrows this technique from two of yoga's warrior poses, in which your pelvis is encouraged to be "squared" (like in a grid) in the same direction for balance and alignment in the spine. Unlock Gridlock also invites you to unlock your hard stare, softening it to create a Drishti (*DRISH-ti*), a point of gaze or focus, which is a yoga technique to create awareness that is attentive but not strained by external stimulation. In Unlock Gridlock, this gaze is Urdhva Drishti (*OORD-vuh DRISH-ti*), a gaze to infinity, helping to organize your concentration, movement, and energy for infinite ease, despite the fact that traffic gridlock can feel like an eternity.

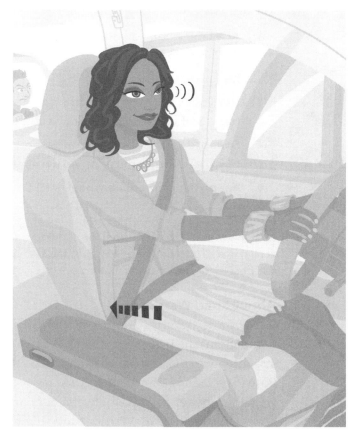

Road Warrior I

strengthen ▪ empower ▪ focus ▪ calm

The wait for the toll bridge is long. You need your inner strength to sit through the wait. Squeeze the steering wheel when it's slow to get a grip on the situation and feel the will of a warrior—strength, focus, and calm under pressure.

Happy-Go-Yoga

HGY Travel Advisory: Do Road Warrior I when traffic is slow, moving only straight forward at a crawl (at the most).

1. At a time when you don't need to turn the wheel, hold the steering wheel at nine o'clock and three o'clock.

2. Keep your elbows bent.

3. Use your back muscles to lower the tops of your shoulders down and back, as if your shoulder blades could move closer together behind you.

4. Squeeze your elbows and upper arm bones toward your ribs, as if you're trying to clutch a purse or file under your arm.

5. Keep your grip on the wheel at all times!

Bonus: For an extra challenge, extend the arms long and maintain the squeezing motion toward the middle, from the shoulders to the arms to the hands on the wheel at all times! (You might need to adjust the seat back at a safe time to do this, and again, this pose is for slow-moving times only.)

About Road Warrior I

Road Warrior I adapts the arm form of a standing pose called Warrior I (Virabhadrasana I: *VEER-uh-buh-DRAHS-uh-nuh*) and combines it with the strengthening of a very challenging, powerful pose called Four-Limbed Staff Pose (Chaturanga Dandasana: *CHAT-ur-AHNG-uh dun-DAHSS-uh-nuh*). In class, we might squeeze a block between our hands to create engagement in the arms and shoulders for Warrior I and squeeze upper arms close to the ribs to strengthen a pretty long list of muscles in Four-Limbed Staff Pose: shoulders, back, upper and lower arms, and chest. In Road Warrior I, the steering wheel is that block and helps create the same kind of endurance against resistance. Since we're trying to find road rage relief, it might seem odd to create more power and endurance while on the road, but the brave warrior (on the road or not) doesn't have to fight all the time. Sometimes, it's about the strength to endure quietly, whether it's at the toll bridge or anywhere else.

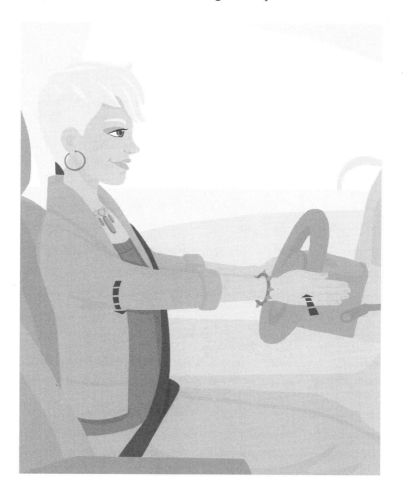

Road Warrior II

relieve ▪ de-stress ▪ empower ▪ calm

Hold on to your steering wheel! Powerless and frazzled, you're hunched over, getting ready to share your aggression with everyone else. Don't yell, flip the bird, or engage in bumper battle. Focus on two spots on your body to find the strength and calm of a warrior, minus the rage.

Happy-Go-Yoga

HGY Travel Advisory: Start when you're stopped or at slow speeds, then maintain for any MPH.

1. Inhale and lift your shoulders as close as you can to your ears. Exhale and let them drop gently.

2. Inhale, lift your shoulders to your ears, and this time, exhale and roll your shoulders toward the seat (your head and body will move back a little), and let them drop gently.

3. Imagine the center of the top of your head lifting to the roof of the car, but keep your chin neutral.

4. Combine steps 2 and 3 more softly and smoothly, matching your shoulder lifts, rolls, and drops to your breathing.

5. Repeat a few times. Sit taller as you relax your neck and widen the front of your chest.

Tip: Do not do this pose while executing a turn. This should be done during a stop or when you're moving straight ahead at slow speeds; then you can keep the position for ultimate benefit throughout the rest of the drive.

About Road Warrior II

Skilled warriors can be peaceful and compassionate, using their minds to overcome opposition without violence. Borrow a technique from the very popular pose Warrior II (Virabhadrasana II: *VEER-uh-buh-DRAHS-uh-nuh*). Road

Warrior II helps your body relax, yet remain alert and not edgy, even if it seems like everything's working against you on this trip. Breathe deeply to calm and relieve your tight neck and shoulders while opening space across the chest to encourage a kinder heart toward other drivers. Virabhadra is the name of a fierce warrior, so don't worry, you'll still be fierce in the right way, when the time is right.

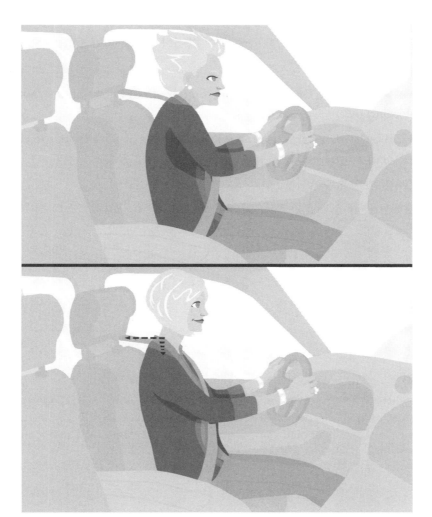

Get Toe'd

relieve ▪ strengthen ▪ refresh

You've finally, finally arrived, and now you need a little pep in your step to get going. Step out of the car to balance your energy and energize your legs and feet. Lock the car door (then check the parking signs carefully so you don't actually get towed). Do this exercise, then proceed to your destination.

Happy-Go-Yoga

HGY Travel Advisory: Do Get Toe'd when you get out of the car and street traffic is not whizzing by.

1. Stand by your car, and use the open door and/or the side of the car for balance, if you need it.

2. Stand on one foot.

3. As you exhale, lift the other knee. Point and flex these toes by moving the ankle.

4. Immediately afterward, put the heel of that foot on the ground, and imagine your toes are windshield wipers. As one unit, wave your toes side to side and let your whole leg rotate at the same time.

5. Switch sides.

Bonus A: During step 4, keep your leg lifted as you wave your toes and rotate the leg for an extra challenge in balance and strength.

Bonus B: You might not even hold on to the car for balance.

Note: If you hear a little pop in your feet and ankles, don't worry. According to the sports medicine specialists at Johns Hopkins University, cracking and popping of joints is usually normal and most of the time is nothing to be concerned about. If something really hurts, though, it's time to ask the doc…what's up?

About Get Toe'd

According to Chinese traditional medicine and many other holistic health practices, when your feet are well, you generally feel energetic and vibrant. Places in the feet correspond to vital organs and tissues in the body. When you do Happy-Go-Yoga's Get Toe'd, you give your feet some extra movement to help the blood circulate, nourishing your entire body through your toes and feet. Get Toe'd is Happy-Go-Yoga's take on a challenging pose called Utthita

Hasta Padangustasana (*oo-TEE-tuh HAHSS-tuh PUH-DUN-goo-STAH-suh-nuh*), which helps create powerful leg muscles as you stand on one foot and lift the other. It also helps you develop better poise and balance, which you might actually need in case your car happens to get t-o-w-e-d. If so, refer to chapter 10, "Global 24/7," to help meditate and let go.

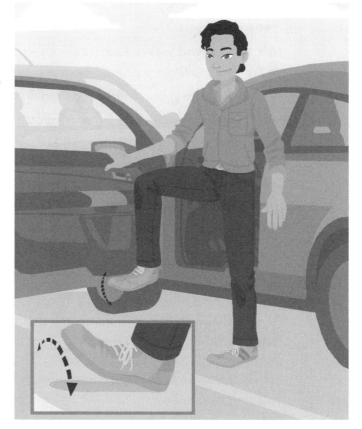

Parking Karma

love ▪ connect ▪ brighten

It's such a bummer to get back to your car and have a ticket because you were just a few minutes too late to catch the parking attendant. Perform this random act of kindness to make someone else's day a lot brighter. Doing something kind will make you feel good, too!

Happy-Go-Yoga

HGY Travel Advisory: Give Parking Karma after you've locked your car, when you're heading toward your destination.

1. Make sure your own meter is paid up.
2. Notice someone else's time about to run out.
3. Put a little spare change into that car's meter and buy that person a little time.
4. If you have a second, leave a nice note on the windshield. It might say "Bought you a little extra time. Pay it forward to someone else next time!"
5. Feel like you did a good deed, smile, and move on with your day.

About Parking Karma

Karma means action—mental, vocal, and physical—from a pure place. In the Western world, we sometimes say, "Oh, that's karma" when we think someone gets what they "deserve," but from the Buddhist perspective, karma is a little bit more like taking noble action based on an opportunity to help in the present, no matter what has happened to you in the past and without expecting something in the future. You might even decide to extend this way of thinking—and your karma—beyond parking and into other parts of your life, too! That's definitely good karma.

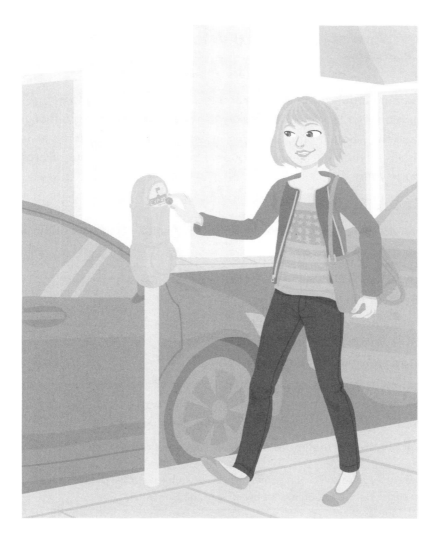

Hey DJ

balance ▪ **de-stress** ▪ **relieve** ▪ **brighten**

You're running around with the kids and the dog in tow, trying to get everything on your list done. "Welcome to the Jungle" is blaring out of your car stereo, and the whole moment is bringing you to your knees. Here's an idea: Have a glam DJ moment to find emotional balance. Change your environment, and change your mood.

Happy-Go-Yoga

HGY Travel Advisory: Do Hey DJ anytime you can safely change your music and keep your eyes on the road.

1. Keep paying attention to the road ahead.

2. Reach for the stereo.

   Option A: If you're listening to the radio, change the station or the music genre. Avoid heavy metal, hard rock, or angry rap. (Depressing lyrics are good to avoid in this moment, too.)

   Option B: If you're listening to music on your connected device, change the song and listen to your favorite bouncy pop or R&B jam, uplifting Broadway tune, or regal and powerful classical piece.

3. Sing, hum, and feel more sane and balanced right away.

Tip: Make sure you're still driving safely as you search for songs, please. Better yet, have your passenger be the DJ, unless it's the dog in the front seat.

About Hey DJ

According to Ayurveda, the five-thousand-year-old sister science to yoga, you can use sound to balance your mood.

- If you're in a heated, tense situation or the summer weather is scorching, choose music that decreases that hotheaded feeling (because that's ultimately bad for everyone while you're behind the wheel).

- If your energy is dragging or your wipers can't keep up with the winter rain, don't choose music that's somber. You'll be fully bummed out by the time you reach your destination.

By the way, when you hum or sing along, you are healing yourself from within. According to health professionals who use sound as therapy, you actually stimulate some vital organs and part of the inner ear that can help improve balance, posture, and ease of movement. Hear, hear!

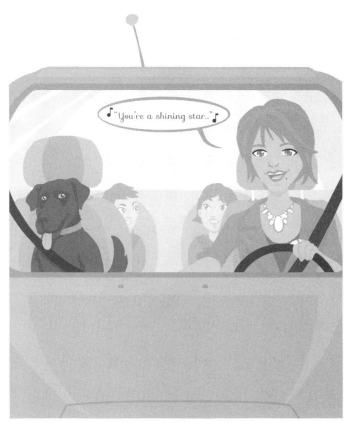

chapter five

Chill, Homies

Home "work" to strengthen and chill out before, during, and after housework

If you're like me, your home is your sanctuary, where you can relax, rest, and nestle in comfort—right? Except, there's that little issue of needing to maintain your cozy nest. Washing dishes and vacuuming dog hair can feel so mundane. I dread ironing.

Here are a few ways to make chores less of a chore and convert them into movement that matters for the body and mind. And, because I'm a big supporter of giving yourself downtime, too, I've included a few things to help us homebodies relax after household tasks, dealing with challenging kids, or finally getting home after an exhausting day running around town. So…chill, homies. Care for home sweet home and care for yourself, too.

In this chapter:

Dive Right In ▪ **Dish It** ▪ **Surf It** ▪ **Garden with the Gods** ▪ **Laundry Lift**
Superhero ▪ **Towel Glide** ▪ **Smartphone Siesta** ▪ **Couch Potato** ▪ **X-tra R&R**

Dive Right In

strengthen ▪ **empower** ▪ **inspire** ▪ **refresh**

You are procrastinating. You have a bunch of stuff to do around the house, and chores have never been your strong suit. Assume the position of an adventuresome diver, ready to take the plunge and get submerged in efficiency. Think of how good you'll feel when you eventually come up for air.

Happy-Go-Yoga

1. Stand with your feet together, toes and heels touching.
2. Place your hands on your hips.
3. Hinge at your hips and fold your upper body over to make a ninety-degree L-shape (as you fold, firm your navel, like you are just trying to keep your belly lifted into your body as you descend).
4. Try to lengthen your spine by reaching the middle of your chest and the top of your head in the opposite direction of your rear end.
5. Reach backward with your hands toward your hips and imagine you have wings.
6. Feel your outer hips wrapping around toward your inner thighs and your inner thighs rolling toward each other and backward through your legs.

   Option A: With your palms facing down, stretch your hands back past your hips.

   Option B: Keep everything the way it is, including the hands reaching back (option A), and rise up onto the balls of your feet.

Tips:

Lower degree of difficulty: Make less of the L shape (keep the chest up higher, place hands on your shins or thighs).

Higher degree of difficulty: Go deeper than the L shape (dive the chest lower toward the feet and lift your heels more).

About Dive Right In

Dive Right In is based on a non-traditional pose, Diver's Pose, and the very traditional, Half Forward Fold (Ardha Uttanasana: *ARD-uh OOT-uh-NAH-suh-nuh*), both of which help yogis prepare for more intricate and challenging poses that require balance and core strength. As you fold yourself in half, your core is fired up to protect your back, and your back muscles are activated to stabilize and lengthen your spine. Your feet, calves, and ankles are working together to keep you in balance as your weight shifts, while muscles in your rear end secure the connection between your upper and lower body. Meanwhile, your shoulders get a stretch as you reach back with your fingers, opening up your chest a little. So don't hesitate. Just dive right in. Even if the list of chores is really long, once you're done, you'll surface, breathe, and be ready to dive right into something much more fun.

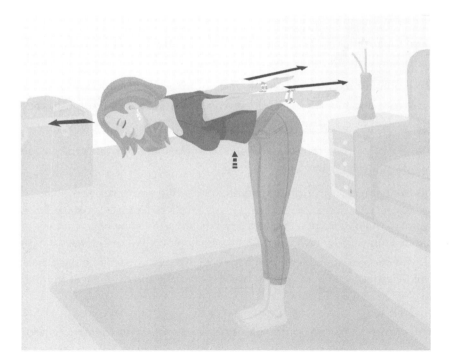

Dish It

strengthen ▪ empower ▪ balance

A pile of dirty dishes in the sink is never fun, but you've got to get through them. Do this pose to help your tummy digest your meal with ease and clear the sink, too.

Happy-Go-Yoga

1. Stand at the sink with your feet separated about hip width apart for stability.
2. As you stand close to the counter and sink area, let your belly lean into the sink counter, but not too much.
3. Inhale through the nose and inflate your belly (you should feel it pressing against the counter a little).
4. Exhale and draw the entire belly into your body and away from the sink counter, without moving anything else.
5. Still on your exhale, imagine lifting your belly button up and in, as if you're trying to tuck it up under your ribs and lock up your midsection.
6. Try to stay relaxed as you suspend your breath.
7. Take a big inhale to release the lock, and exhale normally to release everything.
8. Repeat steps 3 through 7 several times while you scrub the dishes.

Tip: Try not to "hold" your breath out as you exhale, but imagine really pressing out your breath, emptying yourself fully with the movement of the belly inward and up.

Note: Some people experience light-headedness with this pose (it's more powerful than it might seem), so if that happens, breathe normally and try again at another time.

About Dish It

Dish It strengthens the abdominal muscles and massages the organs around the middle of the body. It's a lighter version of a pretty intense yoga lock, or seal, called Abdominal Lock (Uddiyana Bandha: *OO-dee-YAH-nah BAHN-duh*), meant to improve digestion and elimination. Dish It also helps increase circulation, support digestion, and promotes a strong metabolism. Plus, anything that helps the core supports the lower back, too. In an ancient Hatha yoga text called the *Gheranda Samhita*, it's said this lock "destroys decay and death." Like I said, Dish It is a lighter version, so let's just call it Happy-Go-Yoga's way of fitting stealth abdominal toning and internal cleansing into the mix as you clean up the kitchen.

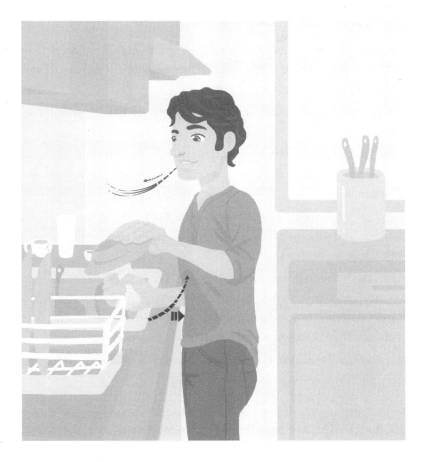

Surf It

strengthen ▪ **brighten** ▪ **balance** ▪ **refresh**

Dust bunnies multiply and float across the floor, and you notice that the carpet is oddly…crunchy. You can no longer put off vacuuming. Drag. If you put a little rolling wave motion into your movement as you roll the vacuum across the floor, then it's a little more like a day at the beach. (Okay, maybe that's an exaggeration, but it's better than just vacuuming.)

Happy-Go-Yoga

1. Place your feet about two or three feet apart while holding on to the vacuum with your hand (the vacuum will be slightly in front of you and to the side, to begin).

2. Step solidly into both feet to feel your center of gravity—strong in the middle.

3. As you pull the vacuum closer to you, shift backward and bend your back knee, putting most of your weight on the leg that's farthest away from the vacuum).

4. If you can, while solidly weighted on the back leg, lift the toes of your front foot and flex them toward your ankle. Dig the heel into the floor a little more firmly for stability.

5. As you push the vacuum away from you, press your back foot into the floor, lengthen that back leg, and use the strength of the back leg to propel your weight forward, into your front leg and over your front foot. Bend your front knee to accommodate the motion.

6. Repeat steps 3 through 5 and get a sense of a smooth rocking motion as you slide the vacuum back and forth.

Bonus: As you get more proficient with Surf It, you'll be able to move around the floor by lifting the back foot on step 5 and replacing the foot in a different location so the rocking motion never stops, just like ocean waves.

About Surf It

Think of waves rolling ashore and back out to sea: There's a calming, rocking quality to them. You can bring a little tranquility to the noisy task of vacuuming with Surf It, which is a standing version of Pose of the War God (Skandasana: *skahn-DAHSS-uh-nuh*), moving into a light Warrior II (Virabhadrasana II: *VEER-uh-buh-DRAH-suh-nuh*).

This pose helps steady your core and strengthen your leg muscles, which help us stand and move through our day. Surf It also stretches the hamstrings and calves while helping you work on your balance. Hopefully, as you dream of surfing the waves in a tropical place, vacuuming will be more of a breeze.

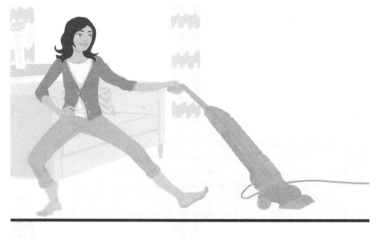

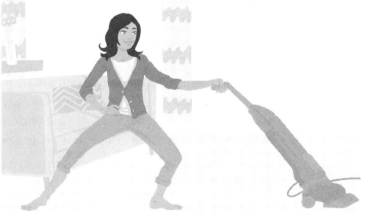

Garden with the Gods

strengthen ▪ empower ▪ inspire ▪ brighten

Your normal green thumb efforts need a little inspiration as you dig up weeds and nourish the soil. It's looking a little wimpy and sad in the garden, and those newly planted seeds need to sprout. Divine intervention couldn't hurt. Might be time to Garden with the Gods.

Happy-Go-Yoga

1. In the garden, on a soft surface like soil or grass, kneel with your toes underneath your rear end.

2. Two options for toes:

   Option A, Tuck: Tuck your toes under and let the balls of your feet touch the ground, like you're making toe prints in the earth, to stretch out the arches of your feet.

   Option B, Untuck: Let your toenails touch the earth to stretch the tops of your feet.

3. Reach your arms up overhead and interlace your fingers, pressing your palms together. (Try to lengthen your arms as much as possible toward the sky, your upper arms framing your ears.)

4. Keeping the fingers interlaced and the palms touching, release your thumb and index finger and press them together while pointing them skyward, as if you could send out a thunderbolt from the tips of your index fingers with your concentration and energy.

5. Keep sitting deeply toward the earth; as you inhale, reach higher toward the sky without lifting your rear.

6. Keep the lift, and exhale while sending energy into the roots of everything in your garden and into your feet as they help nourish your efforts to grow.

7. Repeat steps 5 and 6 until you and your garden are sufficiently inspired (or your thunderbolt arms need a break).

Tip: If you have sensitive knees, try putting a cushion underneath your knees or a thin blanket in between the backs of your thighs and your calves.

About Garden with the Gods

Set aside your shovel for a sec, in favor of a thunderbolt, the weapon of the sky gods. Garden with the Gods is based on yoga's Thunderbolt Pose (Vajrasana: *vaj-RAH-suh-nuh*). It helps strengthen your calf muscles while stretching the arches or the tops of your feet. It can also help improve your posture as you try to center your spine over your pelvis and your pelvis over your feet. You'll also feel this pose in your shoulders, biceps, and upper back the longer you keep them firm and skyward. Garden with the Gods can help encourage meditation and deep breathing, which will likely help you as you finish your weeding.

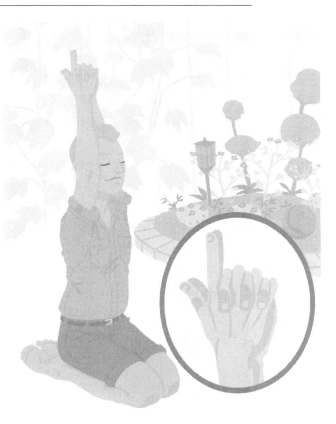

Laundry Lift

strengthen ▪ balance

Is it your imagination or is this laundry basket a lot heavier than the last time you did a load? Are your arms just tired? Lift your laundry using the bigger muscles in your lower body for more power and stability.

Happy-Go-Yoga

1. Look at your laundry basket on the floor and separate your feet in one of two ways: just more than shoulder width apart if your basket is on the narrow side, or wider than shoulder width apart if the basket is a little bigger.

2. Bend your knees and squat down deeply to bring your rear end closer to the floor, but keep your chest up as much as possible. If you can, squat deeper.

3. Feel your center of gravity at your core and breathe deeply.

4. Inhale to prepare as you grab hold of the basket, keeping your heart above the level of your rear end.

5. As you exhale, from the strength of your legs, press your feet into the ground to rise up with the laundry basket.

6. Proceed to the washing machine and refocus your efforts on not mixing the colors and whites.

Tip: If the initial squat, step 2, is a bit too much, bend over a little, grab the basket for stability, then bend your knees into the squat as deeply as you can to bring the rear end lower than the heart. Then, press up with your legs and lift the basket.

About Laundry Lift

Many people hurt their backs doing everyday tasks, especially lifting, by asking vulnerable parts of the body to do too much. Let your stronger parts do the heavy lifting, as they were designed to do. At the same time, strengthen some key muscle groups. Happy-Go-Yoga's Laundry Lift draws upon the benefits of Goddess Pose, or Utkata Konasana (*oot-KAH-tuh koh-NAHSS-uh-nuh*), excellent for building strength in the legs. At the same time, using Laundry Lift to pick up a heavy load—or anything else—will help protect your back, too. (Watch Olympic weight lifters. They use their legs!) Not a bad deal to have all of that know-how to lift things, plus clean clothes. Now, breathe in the scent of clean laundry, and try to meditate while you sort the socks.

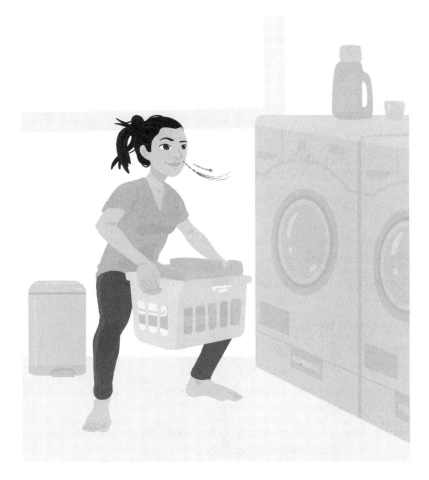

Superhero

inspire · strengthen · relax · love

Cleaning, cooking, and helping with homework…it's all done! You got through all your tasks with speed, agility, and power! Seriously, you feel like a superhero. Let this pose rescue your tired body and spirit, then get some well-deserved rest and relaxation, recharging for the next mission.

Happy-Go-Yoga

1. On a soft surface, such as an evenly folded blanket, sit on your heels, with your shins on the floor.

2. Let the tops of your feet and toenails touch the floor.

   To support your knees: Place an evenly folded blanket between the backs of your thighs and your calves.

   To support your ankles: Place part of a blanket between your ankles and the floor, rolling or folding it to make a long, small pillow.

3. Keep your knees on the floor, close together as you stay seated on your heels.

4. Lean back and walk your hands back so they are under your shoulders and your chest faces upward.

5. Let your fingers point outward (your right hand will turn clockwise and your left hand will turn counterclockwise).

6. Lift your heart toward the ceiling.

7. Press into the floor to help lift your heart and widen the space across the front of your chest.

8. If your neck feels fine, you might try to lean your head back and open the space of your throat.

9. Breathe deeply for three to five breaths before you come down.

10. Repeat steps 6 through 9 twice more, if you like.

Bonus: For more of a challenge, during step 6, lift your rear end off your heels and press your hips and heart upward.

Note: Superhero can be challenging for your knees and ankles, so don't force it. Try the options in step 2, and if something is still bothersome, go directly to the shower and try Towel Glide (page 88).

About Superhero

Superhero is the Happy-Go-Yoga combo of two classic yoga poses: Hero Pose (Virasana: *veer-AH-suh-nuh*) and Upward Plank Pose (Purvottanasana: *pur-voh-tuh-NAH-suh-nuh*). Just like you multitask at home, Superhero accomplishes a bunch of things at the same time. It stretches your thighs, knees, arches, and ankles after all that hard work at home. It's also uplifting for your heart as you stretch the fronts of your shoulders and chest muscles, while relieving tummy tension to improve digestion and dissolving hip tightness. If this pose is practiced regularly, some benefits might include reducing high blood pressure and relieving asthma symptoms. Clearly, this pose has some extraordinary powers to help us. Call upon it anytime you need assistance!

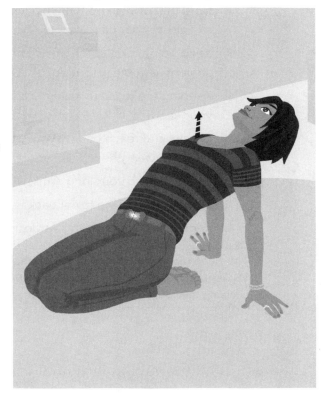

Towel Glide

relieve · relax

That hot shower did you some good. You're a lot more relaxed, but a little more relief for your neck and shoulders would be so welcome. Take advantage of your body's warm temperature post-shower to give yourself a good stretch and a deeper chill-out. Dry off with your towel, then use it for this pose.

Happy-Go-Yoga

1. Dry off after the shower. Put on a soft, loose shirt to keep your body warm.

2. Hold the towel in front of you, lengthwise (and bunch it up in your hands to hold it). Your hands should be about three to four feet apart.

3. Keep holding on to the towel and lengthen your arms in front of you, as straight as you can (but don't lock out or hyperextend your elbows).

4. Keeping the towel taut, inhale and raise your arms and the towel above your head.

5. Exhale, and reach behind you with the towel, keeping the towel taut and your arms lengthened. Let your shoulders drop down your back.

6. Inhale to raise your long arms, with taut towel, above your head again.

7. Exhale to bring the towel back in front of you.

8. Repeat steps 4 through 7 as desired.

Tip: Keep the bathroom warm with the shower's steam or heat to retain suppleness in your body while you do Towel Glide, rather than opening the bathroom door and allowing the cool air to stiffen your softened muscles.

About Towel Glide

Happy-Go-Yoga's Towel Glide is an adaptation of a beloved yoga strap method to benefit some big muscle groups that support arm and upper-body movements every single day. As you bring the towel above your head while holding it taut, you get a stretch on the underside of the arms and in the rib cage muscles. As you bring the towel behind your back and continue to tug it taut, you'll melt away tension in the shoulders and chest. The entire motion relieves tightness in your neck, while pulling the towel uses several muscles in your arms. Keep in mind that Towel Glide is made for normal-sized bath towels. It's not going to work as well if you have those massive sheetlike bath towels. If that's the case, lucky you, but grab a thinner towel instead and prepare to do Laundry Lift (see page 84) the next time your heavier, luxurious towels need to be washed.

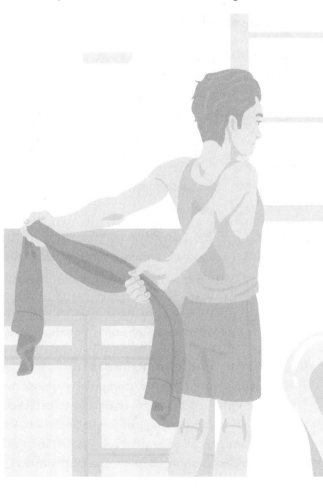

Smartphone Siesta

relieve ▪ relax ▪ calm ▪ empower

Seriously. Stop checking your smartphone every two seconds like an itch you can't stop scratching. Restrain yourself, and consider taking a self-imposed Smartphone Siesta instead. People around the world who take siestas regularly seem to be pretty relaxed and happy, don't they?

Happy-Go-Yoga

1. Sit on your couch. Kick off your shoes. Wiggle your toes.
2. Take your phone in both hands and put it behind your head.
3. Rest the back of your head on the phone, preferably with a pillow in between the phone and your head.
4. Relax your shoulders.
5. Lean back, and widen your elbows.
6. Close your eyes.
7. Inhale smoothly through your nose.
8. Exhale, and make an *mmm* sound, like a bee.
9. Keep the phone behind your head and repeat steps 7 and 8 at least ten times.

Tip: Let the *mmm* sound come more from your gut and not your throat.

About Smartphone Siesta

Even if you don't feel particularly stressed, constantly staring into a small screen with endless amounts of data is registered by your body and mind as a form of effort, and even stress. Happy-Go-Yoga's Smartphone Siesta combines part of a pose called Supported Headstand (Salamba Sirsasana: *suh-LAHM-buh shrr-SHAH-suh-nuh*) with one of the most calming breathing techniques in all of yoga. You're not going to do a headstand in this pose, but the arm shape you use to keep the phone behind your head is a wider version of the base of a supported headstand. In yoga, Headstand is among the more grounding ways of going upside down. The *mmm* sound is part of Bee Breath (Brahmari Pranayama: *BRAH-muh-ree PRAH-nuh-YAH-muh*), meant to calm and pacify despite external noise. You get physical relief with the stretch across your chest and upper back as your elbows reach wider. The more you hum, the deeper you'll go into relaxation. That empowered feeling? It comes from making the choice to break from your smartphone and chill out instead.

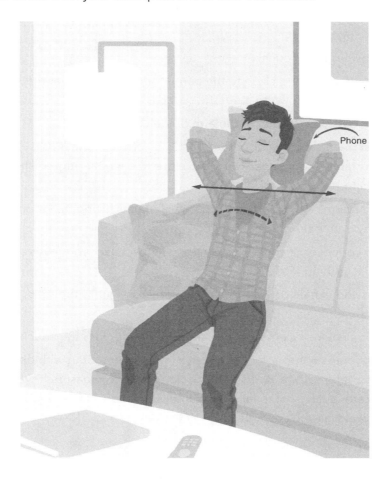

Couch Potato

de-stress ▪ relax ▪ relieve

It's all you want right now...to curl up on the couch and be a potato. The remote is in your hand, but stop. That cop show, reality cooking competition, or political thriller can wait for a Happy-Go-Yoga moment of total relaxation before you stimulate your brain all over again. Best part? You don't even have to get off the couch.

Happy-Go-Yoga

1. Lie down on the couch.
2. Scoot your rear end close to the corner of the couch (near the spot where the arm comes down to meet the seat cushion).
3. Gently toss your legs over the arm of the couch.
4. Adjust the distance of your rear from the corner so that this is comfortable. (Your knees will bend close to a ninety-degree angle, but not quite.)
5. Let your arms rest along your sides, with palms facing up, or on your tummy, with palms facing down.
6. Close your eyes. If you'd like, lay a small towel over your eyes so there's no light coming into them.
7. Inhale and exhale deeply, freeing your mind of junky thoughts each time you exhale.
8. Imagine you're a dense potato, and sink deeper into the couch.
9. Repeat steps 6 through 8 for about three minutes. Start with one minute if three seems like a lot. In fact, you don't have to measure how long you stay here, but try not to fall asleep in this position. Stay a tiny bit aware and awake as you rest and let go of the day.

Bonus: Lie on the carpet or rug (or put a blanket down) with your rear very close to the corner where the wall and floor meet. Put your legs up the wall, making close to an L shape with your body. Lay your arms alongside your body with your palms up.

About Couch Potato

Believe it: It takes a good amount of effort to let your body and mind fully release. Happy-Go-Yoga's Couch Potato is adapted from a classic Restorative yoga pose known as Legs Up The Wall (Viparita Karani: *VEE-puh-REE-tuh kuh-RON-ee*). Couch Potato helps circulation, relieves tired or cramped legs and feet, and relieves tightness in your hips and lower back. It can also release the back of your neck and calm your mind. Restorative yoga is all about setting up the circumstances and environment to relieve the body of tension and restore energy. In this case, your comfy couch will do just fine.

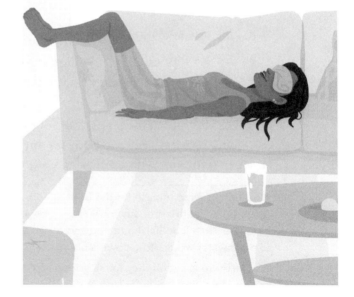

X-tra R&R

relieve ▪ relax

Now that you've done the work to make your home cozy, clean, and comfortable, you need an ultimate way to chill. Lie on your bed, a blanket, or your newly clean carpet and unwind by sprawling out into a big X shape. X-actly what you deserve.

Happy-Go-Yoga

1. Lie down. Inhale and exhale deeply a few times to get comfortable.

2. Inhale. Then exhale and hug yourself into a little ball, hugging your knees to your chin and chest.

3. While still in the ball, inhale easily.

4. Exhale, and release the entire body, letting your arms and legs make an X shape.

5. Inhale easily through the nose.

6. Exhale through your mouth with a big sigh.

7. Repeat steps 2 through 6 a few times as needed to feel like you're melting into the floor.

8. As you repeat the steps, feel your muscles and bones getting heavier. As you breathe, scan the body for any areas where you are holding tension or gripping. With each exhale, sigh out the tension and soften everything.

Bonus: For extra release for the front of your hips, put a firm, thin pillow or evenly folded blanket underneath your pelvis (not your lower back), and let the middle of your body be like a little hill. Imagine every bit of tension flowing out of your hands and feet like rainwater would flow down a hill.

Note: There is a tendency to fall asleep in X-tra R&R, so if you really need to get a good night's sleep, get ready for bed and do this pose to drift off into a deep sleep.

About X-tra R&R

There's a difference between chilling out and *really* chilling out. A Yin yoga pose called Pentacle is the inspiration for Happy-Go-Yoga's X-tra R&R. By making an X shape with the body, and pairing it with specific, extra-relieving inhales and exhales, you allow your limbs and torso to fully relax. It only gets better if your mind can let go, too. X-tra R&R gently stretches the tissues that form joints. This pose is not about stretching tight muscles, but about being receptive to letting the body rehabilitate its hardworking cells and organs.

In other words, X-tra R&R is like giving your body the break it deserves, and that's just X-cellent for your health, period.

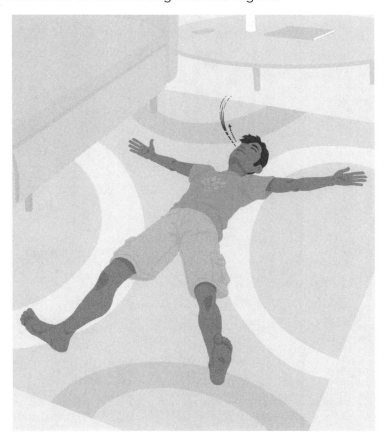

chapter six

Sunny-Side Up

Fresh ways to kick-start the day on the sunnier side of life

Don't you love it when your eyes open and you feel rested and ready for the day? Morning people, this stuff comes naturally for you, but for those of us a little slower to get going, here are a few handy ways to set the day in motion with a sense of positivity and productivity (morning people, you can still benefit, too). One of the most precious times for yogis is when we wake up, which gives us an opportunity to meditate in quiet, set intentions, and create positive thoughts for the day before life's daily challenges start to test us. So greet the light, and start the day right. Hey, I love a good cup of coffee, but these daily kick-starters are pretty eye-opening, too!

In this chapter:

Shine On ▪ **Wise Dreamer** ▪ **Flap and Fly** ▪ *V* **is for Verve**

Brush and Breathe ▪ **Rock Your Heart** ▪ **Sunshine Coffee**

Unbreakable You ▪ **Swimmingly** ▪ **Simba**

Shine On

energize ▪ **refresh** ▪ **brighten**

It only takes a second to greet the day and lift your spirits right out of the gate (or the blankets, really). You don't even have to leave the warmth of your bed to feel the sun's optimistic energy flowing through your body as you begin to move for the first moments of the day.

Happy-Go-Yoga

1. Sit up in bed. (Yes, go ahead and yawn. Your legs will probably feel best if they're in a cross-legged seat.)

2. As you inhale smoothly and fully, stretch your arms upward, as if you were reaching for an imaginary sky and sun in your bedroom. (If your neck feels okay, lift your gaze and lean your head back.)

3. As you exhale, pull your belly button into yourself and bow over your legs.

4. Inhale and stretch your arms forward as far as you can. Slide them down toward the bottom of the bed. Let your head relax.

5. Exhale, pull your belly button in, and begin the cycle again to sit up and reach upward, and inhale to start step 2 again. (If it helps, you can walk your hands closer toward you to sit up again.)

6. Try three times to begin, working up to eight, or as many as you'd like.

Tip: Think of your arms reaching out from the middle of your heart, as if they were an extension of your heart, to feel deeper stretches in your body.

About Shine On

Shine On is born from one of the staples of yoga: Sun Salutation (Surya Namaskar: *SOOR-ee-uh nuh-muh-SKAR*), considered a total body and mind awakener. Traditionally, yogis do 108 Sun Salutations, especially at auspicious times, such as the winter or summer solstices, to honor a sacred number tied to ancient rituals. We use just the arms in the Happy-Go-Yoga version, and do a few simple rounds to get energized for the day.

As you reach up from the heart, you welcome the light of a new day, giving your chest and lungs more space to let oxygen in and fuel your cells. You also stretch your shoulders, which could feel a little cramped from a weird pillow arrangement while you slept. As you fold over the covers and onto the bed, you turn inward toward the heart while activating your core and stretching out your upper back and shoulders. Cycling back to the beginning, you complete one round of saluting the sun and acknowledge the cycle of your beautiful life. If that's not a great way to start the day, what is?

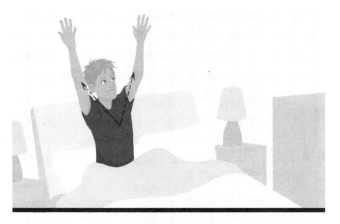

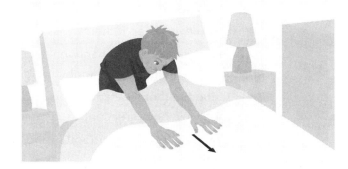

Wise Dreamer

focus ▪ inspire ▪ refresh ▪ relieve

Oh, what was that awesome dream you just had? Sometimes the dream world is so good, you'd like to just stay in it! Or sometimes the dream is a little bit of a nightmare, and you need a moment to let it go. Here's a way to balance your mental energies, either by letting go or by tapping into the mind's power to realize your dreams. Do this as you wake up, or at any time throughout your day when your mind needs refreshing.

Happy-Go-Yoga

1. Sit up tall and take a few deep breaths, matching the duration of your inhale to your exhale (in the morning, this usually means paying a little more attention to your inhale).

2. Choose the appropriate thumb for how you're starting the day: right thumb if you loved the spark of your dreams; left thumb if you need to soothe yourself and let go.

3. Place the thumb in between your eyebrows, but a little higher, on your "third eye." Keep it there.

4. Place your opposite hand, palm up, on your thigh (same side as that hand), and join your thumb and forefinger at the finger pads.

5. Using the thumb at your brow, rub gently and slowly in a small, circular motion in one direction, keeping the thumb connected to your skin.

6. Continue breathing smoothly and deeply. Try not to count the number of times you make a circle.

7. Repeat step 5, switching the direction of the circle as you massage your third eye. Stay with the same thumb, and keep your thumb on your skin.

Note: Your intuition will tell you when it's time to switch directions in step 7, and also when to stop.

About Wise Dreamer

Your third eye is the focal point of Happy-Go-Yoga's Wise Dreamer. The ancient yogis believed the third eye was the energetic location of dreams, intuition, wisdom, and knowledge. It's the place where your yoga practice and the transformation that comes with it come together in the system of the chakras (*CHUH-kruhz*), the subtle energies of the body. By using your left thumb, you'll channel your more quiet, feminine, and grounded energies. With your right thumb, you fire up the more assertive, masculine energies. With your bottom hand, you'll make Jnana mudra (*GYAHN-uh MOO-druh*), a gesture of wisdom and clarity. Stimulating and soothing the energetic space of the third eye can help you release what's stuck, unleashing potential—the great awakening we all dream about.

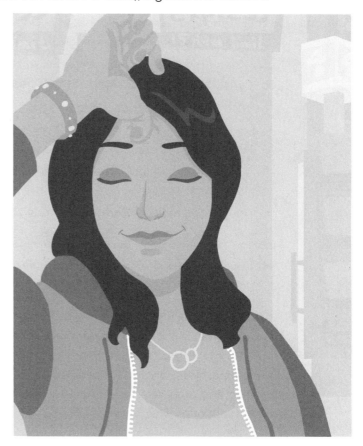

Flap and Fly

brighten ▪ refresh ▪ strengthen

It's one of those mornings. You woke up on the wrong side of the bed and don't want to get up and face the day. Flip your mood with quick flips of the wrist to shake it off and feel a little more uplifted.

Happy-Go-Yoga

1. Stand with your feet about hip or shoulder width apart.

2. Extend your arms out so that your body makes a T shape. (Try to keep your shoulders from creeping up.)

3. Keeping your shoulders and arms stable and strong, start to think of your wrists and hands feeling loose and flexible.

4. With your fingers loose, begin to flap your hands at the wrists, still keeping your shoulders down and your arms firm from the shoulders to the wrists.

5. Let your fingers and hands go completely to do whatever they're going to do as they flap.

6. Inhale and exhale deeply at a steady pace for ten breaths to start.

Tip: Firm your whole body; the only parts that move are your wrists, hands, and fingers.

Note: The longer you do Flap and Fly, the more your shoulders and arms might start to fatigue, so steady your breath to create more endurance and power.

About Flap and Fly

Happy-Go-Yoga's Flap and Fly gets harder the longer you do it! The longer you hold your shoulders and arms steady, the more you work the shoulder, back, and arm muscles. Flap and Fly is based on a Kundalini yoga kriya (*KREE-yuh*), a method and practice focused on a specific result or a physical movement to connect with one's flow of energy. Flap and Fly is a balance of holding steady and strong (arms and shoulders) while letting go of control (wrists, hands, and fingers), which can often relieve us of attachment and suffering. As you flap the hands, the movement from the wrists out is like shaking out the negative feelings that might be bringing you down. Get rid of them to feel light enough to fly. Plus, if you think Flap and Fly is kind of silly, you might be surprised by a spontaneous smile. There. Mood flipped. Proceed with day, please.

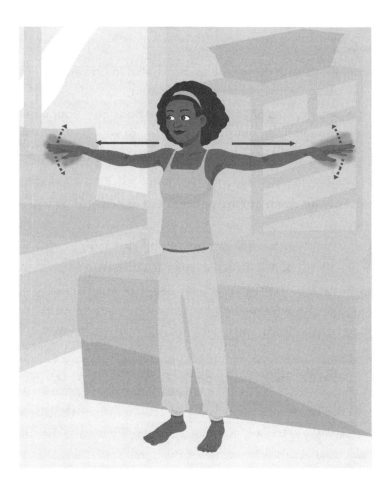

V is for Verve

relieve ▪ refresh ▪ calm ▪ strengthen

You roll out of bed, and you're really dragging. You know you're going to need every bit of energy for the busy day ahead. Try this pose to spark verve, vigor, and vitality! V. exciting!*

(*V. = very)

Happy-Go-Yoga

1. Step your feet about three feet apart, parallel to one another (if you're a really tall person with long legs, farther apart).
2. Press the outer edges of your feet into the floor. Feel your inner ankles lift up away from the floor, but still keep all ten of your toes pressing down.
3. Inhale, put your hands on your hips, and lift the center of your chest.
4. Exhale, keep your torso long, and lean forward, hinging at the hips.
5. Try to keep your spine as long and straight as possible as you reach for the floor.
6. Press your hands into the floor right under your shoulders.
7. Inhale and lift up, with your back rather flat.
8. Exhale and start to fold deeper at your hips so that the top of your head starts to reach for the floor.
9. Stay here for thirty seconds to one minute if you can.
10. To stand back up, put your hands on your hips, feel your tailbone get heavy toward the floor, and hinge back up to stand.
11. Step or hop your feet back together.

Tip: If the floor seems very far away, put your hands on your shins to stabilize yourself.

Tip: If your lower back is particularly sensitive, bend your knees very slightly to give it some space.

Bonus A: If the floor is close, put your palms on the floor.

Bonus B: Lower the top of your head (gently) all the way to the floor and walk your hands back to press your palms into the floor in line with your feet. (P.S. This bonus is v. hard!)

About *V* is for Verve

V is for Verve (and vigor, and vitality), which is exactly what you need to start a busy day. Happy-Go-Yoga's version of this pose is a homey take on Wide-Legged Forward Bend (Prasarita Padottanasana: *pra-sa-REE-tah puh-doe-tuh-NAHS-uh-nuh*), a pose that helps counteract fatigue, foggy-headedness,

back stiffness, and mild depression. Physically, it stretches and strengthens your inner and outer legs, lengthens your spine, and stretches your back muscles, which might have that sleepy, cramped feeling. Let's have less of that and more verve, please!

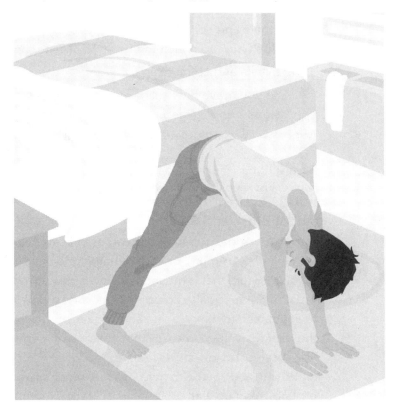

Brush and Breathe

balance • focus • calm • de-stress

You have a lot on your plate today, so you want to start off feeling on top of your game and balanced. Make Brush and Breathe part of your morning routine so that no matter what comes your way, you'll set the tone of steadiness despite challenge. You can get there in the amount of time it takes to brush your teeth.

Happy-Go-Yoga

1. Load up your toothbrush with toothpaste.

2. Inhale and count to six (or eight), brushing at the same time, though you don't have to match the brush strokes to the count.

3. Exhale and count to six (or eight), and continue to brush.

4. As you move the brush around your mouth and across your teeth, repeat steps 2 and 3, keeping the count matching—either six or eight.

5. Continue to Brush and Breathe until you've finished brushing your teeth.

Bonus: If you can breathe a little deeper, go ahead and lengthen the count to ten or twelve; just keep the count even on inhales and exhales.

About Brush and Breathe

Happy-Go-Yoga's Brush and Breathe is based on a tried-and-true pranayama (*PRAH-nuh-YAH-muh*), or yoga breathing technique, called Sama Vritti (*SAH-muh VREE-tee*) that is meant to calm, center, and balance the spirit. Brush and Breathe guides you to combine brushing strokes with a breath count, so you train yourself to make inhale and exhale lengths more equal. You'll support the nervous system in a way that balances the energy you need to do things with a calm and low-stress feeling. You know the phrase "even-keeled"? Count on Brush and Breathe to help you feel more even-keeled, more often. You'll probably end up with more evenly cleaned teeth, too.

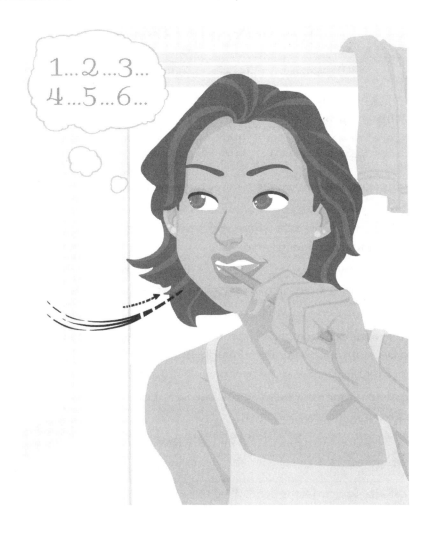

Rock Your Heart

relieve ▪ **balance** ▪ **brighten** ▪ **love**

Your back is kind of creaky, and you're kind of cranky, from a not-so-good night's sleep. Try giving your back some extra love by rocking your heart. You'll get back relief, and who knows, it might make you a little less cranky, too, as you feel the love. You can do this at the breakfast counter, the table, or even just sitting down before you put on your shoes.

Happy-Go-Yoga

1. Find a comfortable seat where you have room to move a little (so don't be close to a table in front you).
2. Sit upright by feeling your sits bones (the large, bony points of the underside of the pelvis) connect with your chair.
3. Put your hands on your hips to stabilize your pelvis and your seat.
4. Inhale and lift the center of your chest upward, feeling the lift come from the back of your heart, or the middle of your upper back between your shoulder blades.
5. Exhale and pull your belly button into your body, fold over a little bit, and tuck your chin into your chest.
6. Repeat steps 4 and 5, as one complete pose, at least five times.
7. Keep going if the groove strikes you to keep rocking your heart.

Tip: Try really hard not to let the bend of the spine be entirely in your lower back; give your lower back much-needed space and love. Think of lifting the front and the back of the heart as you rock.

About Rock Your Heart

Happy-Go-Yoga's Rock Your Heart is based on one of yoga's most beautiful heart openers and backbends, called Camel Pose, or Ustrasana (*oo-STRAH-suh-nuh*), giving it a rockin' dance movement. It simultaneously makes the spine a little less stiff and stretches the area of the chest. Creating more awareness in your heart space allows you to be more compassionate toward yourself (and everyone you see throughout the day). Rock Your Heart also stretches your abdomen and pelvic region in a balanced way, activating the abdominal muscles and nourishing the inner organs with motion to remain healthy and flexible…so rock it.

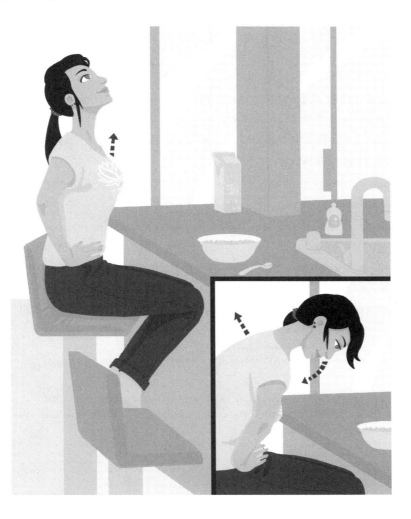

Sunshine Coffee

empower ▪ refresh ▪ brighten

You're still not quite awake, and you're inclined to guzzle your first, second… and maybe your third cup of coffee to clear your foggy mind. Instead, use the power of your breath to wake you up quickly and get you out of that fog. You'll push the cloudiness aside and clear the path for the day ahead.

Happy-Go-Yoga

1. Put down the coffee, if just for a moment.
2. Inhale fully and smoothly through the nose and let the breath expand your belly, midsection, and chest.
3. Pause at the top of the breath, and exhale out through your mouth fully, letting everything go.
4. Close your mouth. Now, swiftly inhale through the nose and expand your belly and midsection just like you did in step 2.
5. Keep your mouth closed. Swiftly exhale through the nose and get rid of as much air as you can, by compressing your abdomen into your body as much as possible to push the air out of your system.
6. Repeat steps 4 and 5, keeping your inhale and exhale swift and powerful. Speed up inhales and exhales, but don't lose the fullness of the breath in or out.

Tip: Use this anytime you normally would grab a cup of coffee for energy throughout the day.

Note: Sunshine Coffee is not for you if you're pregnant or have high blood pressure. If this is you, stick with deep breaths in and out, and keep the pace slow and steady. It'll still be refreshing.

About Sunshine Coffee

Happy-Go-Yoga's Sunshine Coffee is a powerful intake of energy and purge of heaviness in one action, based on Bellows Breath, or Bhastrika Pranayama (*BAH-stree-kuh PRAH-nuh-YAH-muh*). Just like bellows that fan the fire and gives it more force, Sunshine Coffee helps increase your digestive fire by using your abdominal muscles to pump air in and out. By increasing your digestive power, you burn out what is stagnant and unnecessary. The powerful breath is also like a hearty gust of wind, clearing a cloudy mind and invigorating it. The Chopra Center says the metabolic burst from this breath technique can support weight loss. Some experts claim that about coffee, too, but this is the organic way.

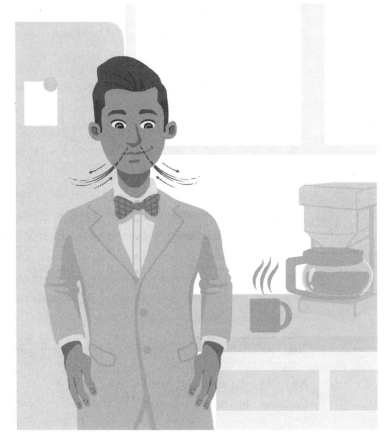

Unbreakable You

empower ▪ **inspire** ▪ **focus**

It's a big day for you, but you're feeling a little less confident than usual. You know you have the skills, and you've prepared for this moment, but you're having some challenges believing in yourself. Strike the pose of unshakeable confidence and trust…in yourself. No one will suspect; they'll only feel your confident energy when you enter the room.

Happy-Go-Yoga

1. Either standing or sitting up, let your shoulders roll back.
2. Lightly place your palms on the solar plexus, right below your chest and right above your belly button.
3. Interlace your fingers and extend your thumbs upward, toward your chest.
4. With your elbows reaching out to the sides of your body, past your ribs, pretend you're trying to pull your hands apart.
5. Let the interlaced fingers form a lock that doesn't allow you to pull your hands apart.
6. As you pull, try not to let your shoulders creep toward your ears; instead, slide your shoulder blades down toward your waist and lift higher through the crown of the head.

Tip: You can do this one anytime you need to connect with your inner strength!

About Unbreakable You

Unbreakable You is based on Unshakeable Confidence and Trust mudra (Vajrapradama mudra: *VAJ-ruh-pruh-DAH-muh MOOD-ruh*), an ancient hand gesture. When you try unsuccessfully to pull apart your hands, it's a symbol that you trust your own will and power, and they can't be broken. Physically, your shoulders and arms feel the resistance, and you work your shoulder, upper back, upper arm, and chest muscles. Simultaneously, Unbreakable You relieves tension in the shoulders and upper back. Hold the mudra at your solar plexus, and it corresponds to the subtle yogic energy of self-confidence and a healthy, non-arrogant ego. We all have those moments when we should trust ourselves a little more. Happy-Go-Yoga's Unbreakable You helps remind you that you can go with your gut and trust it to guide you.

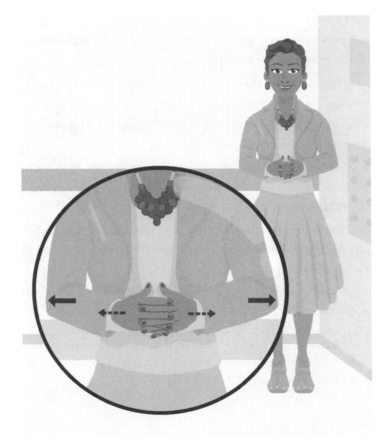

Swimmingly

brighten · love · connect · relieve

Alone. That's kind of how you're feeling today. Rather than hiding from everyone, open up to connect with others and let the day flow. Sometimes it's just a matter of being open to receive, which can help things go a little more smoothly and swimmingly. You never know what each day can bring!

Happy-Go-Yoga

1. Stand with your back against the wall. Feel your feet firmly planted into the floor, about hip width apart.

2. Let your tailbone feel like it's reaching for the floor as it gets support from the wall.

3. Feel your shoulder blades rest against the wall and get a sense of lengthening yourself toward the ceiling.

4. With your forearms and palms near your sides, press them into the wall, connecting solidly to the wall from the fingertips and palms of your hands to the elbows.

5. As you press into the wall, lift just your heart up and away from the wall, letting your shoulder blades move slightly closer together. Keep your rear on the wall.

6. Breathe a little deeper, and each time you inhale, feel the heart lifting up a tiny bit more.

Tip: If you've ever been snorkeling, think of that same body shape as you do this pose, leading with the upper body, reaching back with your feet and lower body while your arms are along your sides.

About Swimmingly

Happy-Go-Yoga's Swimmingly is a vertical version of Fish Pose, or Matsyasana (*MOTZ-ee-AH-suh-nuh*). Think about it—fish are never alone; they're always with their buddies in a school. Swimmingly helps release neck muscles as you stretch your heart up and out of your shoulder area. It opens up tight chest muscles and works your upper back muscles as well. Like a fish, you'll keep flowing through the day, surrounded by pals who are doing the same.

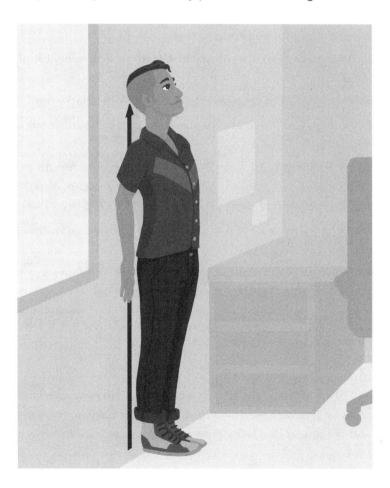

Simba

relieve ▪ empower ▪ inspire ▪ de-stress

As you go about your day, something is already brewing within and ready to burst out of you. Is it frustration? Excess energy? Personal prowess? Either way, put it out there so you can rule the day. Let 'em hear you roar.

Happy-Go-Yoga

1. Stand or sit upright and proud.
2. Take a deep breath in through your nose, then sigh every bit of air out of your body.
3. Prepare by thinking of what you can release from deep within, at the gut.
4. Inhale through your nose and pause at the top of your breath without tension.
5. Exhale forcefully through your mouth, widening your mouth as much as possible, and stick your tongue out as far as you can. And (this is important), at the same time, let out a roaring sound from deep within.
6. Repeat steps 4 and 5 at least once, fully (no wimpy roars…there must be sound).
7. As needed, repeat throughout the day or a few more times in a row to feel your own fire get stoked or released.

Note: You can start at home in private at first, but eventually, feel free to use Simba anytime you'd like to let go and release your power.

About Simba

Lions just kind of know they rule. Happy-Go-Yoga's Simba (aka the Lion King) is based on a powerful pose called Lion Pose or Simhasana (*sim-HAH-suh-nuh*), combined with a popular and hefty energy release practiced in many classes today. When you're holding on to something and just need to let go, Simba helps release tension in the chest and gut. At the same time, it can also inspire more personal power in a single roar. FYI, this is supposed to clean your tongue, freshen your breath, and keep the facial skin firm as you get older. Make some noise about that!

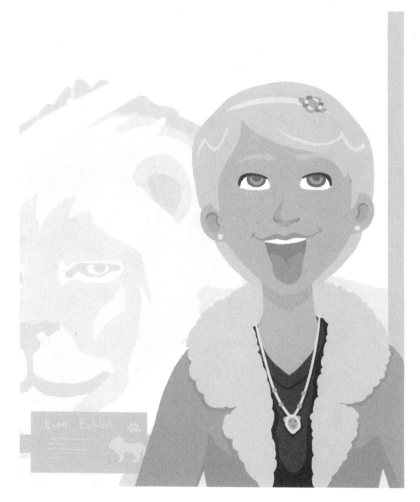

chapter seven

Family Fun

**All-ages activities for more love,
health, and positivity—together**

The family that plays together stays together, don't you think? Today's modern family comes in all shapes, colors, and sizes—unique and full of activities that let us hang out for some good quality time. You can bring a little more happiness and health into the family get-together with poses for watching TV, park picnics, school, camping trips, the aquarium, or the museum. There are even a few in here to help you decompress, because we all know, no matter how much we love our families, there are some not-so-fun moments, too. Kids and adults can do all these poses together. Play and see what happens!

In this chapter:

Slither ▪ **Jaws** ▪ **Mind the Monkey** ▪ **What-EVER!** ▪ **Sprout**
Hug of Joy ▪ **Through the Fire** ▪ **Flipper** ▪ **Picnic Pigeon** ▪ **Love Multiplier**

Slither

brighten ▪ love ▪ strengthen ▪ connect

You're all in front of the TV, watching the family's favorite reality singing competition, but there's a big difference of opinion about who should win. It's getting a little heated. Hmm. Slither to the floor, closer to the TV, so you can tune out the rest of the noise and open your heart to receive all those different opinions, with love.

Happy-Go-Yoga

1. Lie on your belly on a blanket, carpet, or rug with your forehead facing down.
2. Let your toenails and the front of your hips feel the floor, and keep them there.
3. Press your palms into the floor next to your rib cage.
4. Step 3 will automatically bend your elbows—squeeze them close to your body so they are pointed to the ceiling.
5. As you face the TV, imagine that the middle of your chest is being pulled toward it, but your hands, feet, and hips stay right where they are.
6. Inhale, and press into the floor a little more to lift the center of your chest (you don't have to come up a lot). At the same time, try to stretch your toes back a lot without lifting them off the floor.
7. Lift your gaze gently to the TV, but keep your chin tucked in slightly (don't throw your head back a lot).
8. Exhale, and come back down to step 1.
9. Repeat steps 1 through 8 a few times, as you'd like.

Tip: Instead of bending your back to lift your chest and gaze, try to make a smooth arc and lead with your heart. Let your palms feel like they're pulling the floor toward your toes at the same time.

Tip: Start with a small Slither and lift your chest off the ground just a little, then guide it to a slightly bigger Slither, coming up a little higher.

Note: It doesn't matter how high you come off the floor. As your back and legs get stronger, you'll be able to extend your heart up and away!

About Slither

Slither is a version of Cobra Pose, or Bhujangasana (*boo-juhn-GAH-suh-nuh*), a mini backbend in the upper back that helps brighten the heart and strengthen the arms, legs, and back. Slither will help you build more strength and flexibility in the upper and lower arms as well as develop back muscles that can help

support your spine. At the same time, you're stretching chest and shoulder muscles. *Bhujanga* means "serpent." As you lift your head, it's like you're a serpent about to strike. Careful, though— lead with your heart as you lift your head. No need to attack anyone in your family, even if you disagree with who's winning on the show.

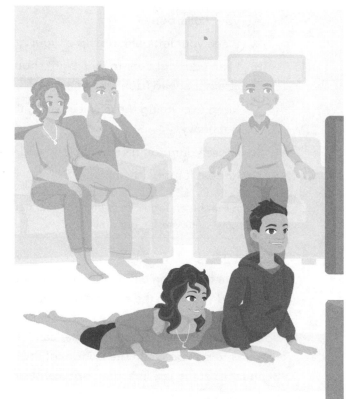

Jaws

relieve • relax • de-stress

School finals have you feeling anxious, and the more you concentrate, the tighter you feel from your brows to your neck. You didn't even realize you were clenching your jaw. Did you know letting go of that grip can help you get a grip on tension overall? Chew on this pose a little and see for yourself.

Happy-Go-Yoga

1. Place your right palm higher on the left side of your chest, right below your collarbone.
2. Place your left palm on top of your right.
3. Lean your right ear to your right shoulder, keeping the face looking straight ahead (don't let it tilt toward your shoulder).
4. Keep everything the way it is; open the mouth slowly and feel your jaw get heavy.
5. Close your mouth without clenching your jaw.
6. Repeat for the other side.

Tip: It might be enough of a stretch for your neck at step 3. If you want to intensify the pose, move on to step 4, but don't force it

About Jaws

There is a muscle on either side of your neck that extends to the top of your chest and shoulder, the sternocleidomastoid, which can get tense with stress. Happy-Go-Yoga's Jaws is one of the simple stretches I use all the time to help loosen these strap-like muscles that can be as tight as a thick rope. When you create the pull between the bottom of the muscle in your chest area and where it attaches at the jaw line, then open and close your mouth to contract and release the muscle, you physically help it to let go of the tightness in your face, shoulders, back, and chest, too—all of which can help you breathe easier. You definitely need that to ace the test later on. Jaws can be good for other tense times, too, when life feels like a test.

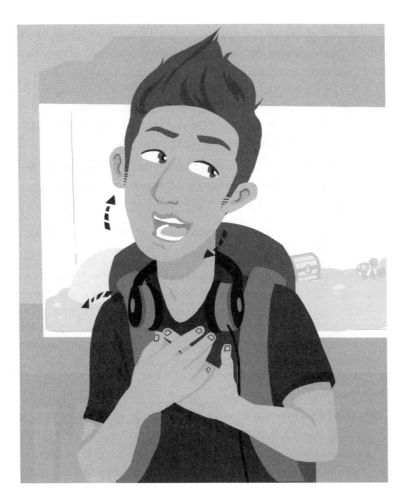

Mind the Monkey

empower ▪ calm ▪ balance

Despite what your super-supportive family members tell you, you're experiencing a wave of self-doubt. You're not like this all the time, but at this moment, it's hard to conquer the voices in your head. Join the club. With this pose, you might feel a little more courageous and discover extraordinary talents you didn't know you had. Go big!

Happy-Go-Yoga

1. Bend your left elbow and keep it near your side while you angle your left palm, facing up, in the area of the right rib cage.
2. Make a fist with your right hand, and put your right elbow in the palm of the left hand. (You'll make a backward L shape with your forearms.)
3. Breathe naturally and relax your shoulders.
4. Imagine you're holding a strong weapon, strong enough to battle your demons.
5. Hold for a minute at first, then, increase to five or more minutes while you breathe calmly and let unwanted thoughts float out of your mind.

Tip: It's best to practice this in a comfortable, seated position, but if you're standing around, there's absolutely no harm in doing this on your feet. That way, you might be more ready to take that leap of faith—who knows?

About Mind the Monkey

In yoga, when your mind jumps around from thought to thought and is a constant stream of worries, lists, and meandering rants, we call it the "monkey mind." The primary reason for practicing yoga is to calm the monkey mind for mental clarity and meditation. Happy-Go-Yoga's Mind the Monkey is based on a hand shape called the Club of Hanuman (Mudgara mudra: *mood-GARR-uh MOO-druh*), featuring the deity Hanuman, a monkey god who took magnificent leaps of faith by shedding self-doubt and inner demons to reveal a giant grace and talent within. In some story versions, his club/weapon is a way to battle those demons inside. You can do this, too! Hanuman is also considered to be very brave and loyal. Do Mind the Monkey with a special friend to seal your friendship and help bring out the best in each other. Also, it's believed this gesture can help stimulate the immune system and fight off illness.

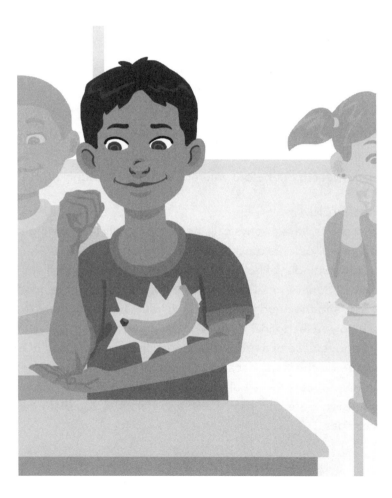

What-EVER!

relieve · de-stress · strengthen

Everyone in your family is just annoying to you right now, for no reason at all. You're mind is spinning, and your shoulders are all bunched up around your ears. You need to let go of the hundred-pound weight on your shoulders. It'll be good for you and for everyone around you.

Happy-Go-Yoga

1. Take a big breath in through your nose as you bring your shoulders to your ears, as far up as they will go.

2. Hold them up for a moment.

3. Let out a big, swift exhale through your nose, and let the shoulders drop swiftly and with some weight.

4. Let all the breath out before you repeat steps 1 through 3.

About What-EVER!

There are few easier ways to physically and emotionally let the weight of the world fall off your shoulders quickly than this little move. Happy-Go-Yoga's What-EVER! is a reminder of how kids shrug their shoulders and let them drop as a way to say "I dunno!" or "Whatever." When you let go of the need to know, the need to do, and the need to figure it out, you have a big, free What-EVER! moment to help you let go in a big way. By lifting and dropping your shoulders you contract and release of a group of muscles that are overused in modern life: the rhomboids, the levator scapulae, and the trapezius. As you release, What-EVER! helps create more balance throughout your upper body and frees a cluster of tension there, too. BTW, it can also help free you of the need for multiple massages.

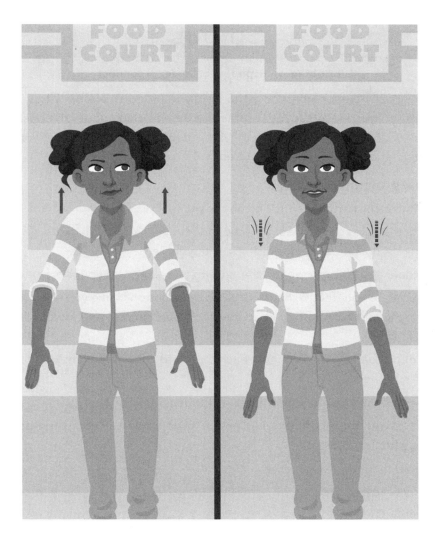

Sprout

brighten ▪ inspire ▪ balance ▪ connect

The family's all here for a barbecue, and while the food smells delicious, you're still a little peeved at your brother for throwing you under the bus. You really want to forgive him, though. Sprout from the muddiness of your misunderstanding and emerge in a better, more enlightened place.

Happy-Go-Yoga

1. Sit in a comfortable spot, like on the grass.
2. Put the soles of your feet together and let your knees fall to the sides gently, making a diamond shape with your legs.
3. Inhale and lift both feet off the ground to balance on your sits bones.
4. Separate your feet, exhale, pull your belly button in like you're trying to hide it, and tuck both of your arms inside and under your knees with the palms up.
5. Keep breathing and connect each thumb to a forefinger, making an "A-OK" hand gesture.
6. Keep balancing on your sits bones (not your tailbone).
7. Keep your belly button pulled in, but lift your heart so your shoulders are as wide as possible.
8. Hold there for five breaths.
9. To come out, untuck your arms first, then lower your legs back into the diamond shape.

Bonus: In Sprout, gaze upward without falling backward, while keeping your feet separated.

Tip: If your hips feel too tight to Sprout, stay in step 2 for a little longer and lean forward (try not to slump) to open up your hips more before moving on to step 3. And, if you stay in step 2, keep breathing.

About Sprout

All at once, Happy-Go-Yoga's Sprout can help ground you, free your positive energy, and open your heart to forgive. It's based on a version of Blossoming Lotus Pose (Vikasitakamalasana: *VEE-kuh-see-TOCK-uh-muh-LAH-suh-nuh*), which helps you unbury dark energy and let go of negativity and blame. Lotus flowers represent our ability to bloom from dark places in our hearts and minds into happier spaces in which we can be more giving and compassionate toward others. In Sprout, balancing on your sits bones relieves hip tightness, strengthens your core, and firms the muscles in the upper back and arms. You literally take the shape of a lotus flower emerging from the murky waters of your past. The "A-OK" hand shape represents wisdom and the knowledge that whatever happened is part of the journey.

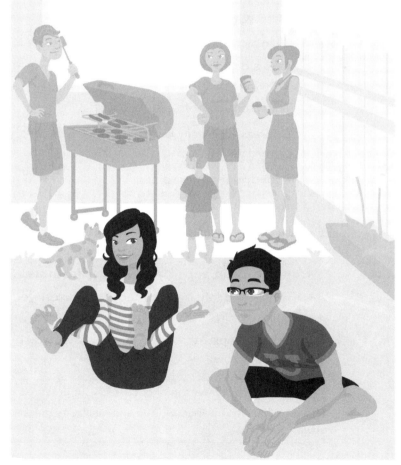

Hug of Joy

love ▪ relax ▪ brighten ▪ refresh

It's been freezing outside for days, and you're cooped up inside the house with your family. There's been a little too much quality time, if you know what I mean. Move in and out of a few joyful hugs to cope with the cold, the cabin fever, and your stir-crazy tendencies right about now.

Happy-Go-Yoga

1. Sit in a chair and make sure your feet are on the floor.
2. Take a big, smooth inhale while you lift your arms up into an open V shape.
3. Take a big, smooth exhale, and:

   ▪ Depress your belly button like you're trying to pull it through your body toward your back;

   ▪ Round your upper spine;

   ▪ Tuck your chin into your chest; and

   ▪ Hug yourself as you fold in, crossing your right arm over your left arm as you fold them into your midsection.

4. Inhale, sit up, and lift your arms up (as in step 2).
5. Exhale and fold in (as in step 3), and cross your left arm over the right in another hug.
6. Repeat steps 2 through 5 several times (you don't have to count, just go with the flow).

Tip: Try not to suck breath in or out; keep your breath as smooth as possible.

Bonus: When you lift your arms up and inhale, try to lift the chin a little and gaze upward.

About Hug of Joy

Specific breathing can help calm the mind and refresh the body's vital functions. The combination of smooth inhaling and exhaling helps your nervous system calm down, settling your cabin fever anxiety. As you move your arms and the torso in Hug of Joy, you'll help blood flow from the center of your chest into your arms and fingers to relieve cold hands. At the same time, you give your body a boost by pumping fresh oxygen through it. The movement also helps alleviate shoulder and chest tightness, which happens when it's cold outside. Hugging yourself over and over is a nice way to stir up more love within, until it gets warm enough to go outside again!

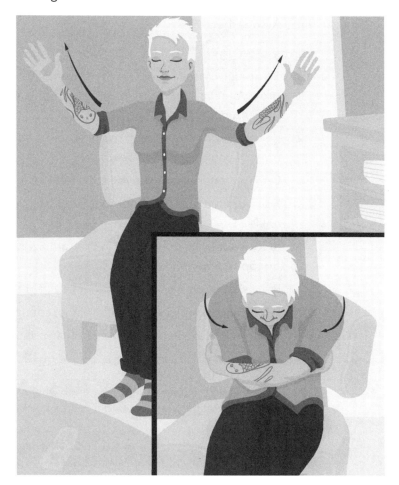

Through the Fire

relieve ▪ empower ▪ inspire

On a family camping trip, you find yourself feeling extra nostalgic and sensitive. Beautiful and powerful memories are resurfacing. Release some of those stored emotions and move into the future, inspired by all that you've been through together.

Happy-Go-Yoga

1. Sit up tall, cross-legged, on the ground. If your lower back is rounded, prop yourself up on a blanket or cushion so your spine lengthens out of the ground.

2. Keeping your knees bent, move your left shin to make a horizontal line in front of you as you look down.

3. Let your left foot's pinkie toe touch the ground.

4. Flex your left foot by bending the ankle, bringing your toes closer to your ankle.

5. Stack your right shin on top in the same way, letting your right ankle be on top of your left knee.

6. Press down—gently—on the top of your right thigh to deepen the stretch.

7. Inhale and exhale for several breaths (count to ten if that helps you).

8. Stretch both legs out in front of you and shake them out.

9. Switch sides and repeat steps 2 through 8.

Tip: To open up your hip more, take your thigh where it meets the hip crease and rotate it outward (clockwise for your right thigh, counterclockwise for your left thigh, before you switch).

Tip: If it's too challenging right now to bend both knees and stack your shins, extend one leg long in front of you and do steps 2–4, one leg at a time.

Note: Don't force the ankle and knee to touch. If your ankles and knees are really far apart, put a folded blanket or pillow between your ankle and knee for padding and supportive spacing.

About Through the Fire

Happy-Go-Yoga's Through the Fire is shaped by the yoga pose Fire Log, (Agnistambhasana: *OGG-nee-stum-BAH-suh-nuh*). When hips are tight, the yogis say we probably have a lot of emotional junk cluttering our bodies and minds, and we're holding on to past experiences that don't necessarily support

our future and growth. Through the Fire helps relieve stress in general, plus it gives you a deep stretch for the outer hips and groin. As you flex your feet, you protect your knees as you go deeper into your thoughts. Keep breathing as you free heavy emotions and invite inspiration.

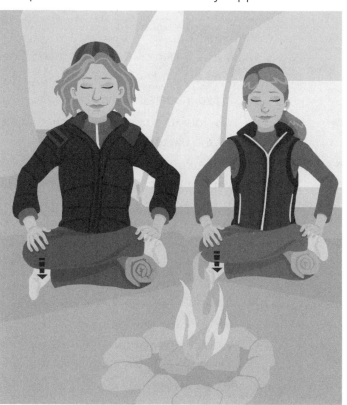

Flipper

strenthen ▪ brighten ▪ connect

It's a beautiful day at the beach with the family, and you're just chillin' behind your shades. At least that's what everyone thinks! Not in the mood to build sand castles, you're toning your body while sitting in your beach chair and smiling like a dolphin. It's your little beach secret (at least for now).

Happy-Go-Yoga

The Legs

1. In your beach chair, lean back and extend your legs, but keep a slight bend in your knees.
2. Dig your heels into the sand.
3. Flex your toes toward your shins evenly, flexing even the pinkie toes, not just the big toes.
4. Without moving in your seat, act like you're dragging your heels to your seat, but don't actually move your heels.

The Arms

1. In your beach chair, lean back and rest your body in the chair.
2. Move your elbows toward the back of the armrests where they meet the chair.
3. Use your upper back muscles to try to hug your upper arm bones toward your body without moving them off the armrest.
4. Without moving your forearms, feel the tiniest rotation of the upper arm bones—your whole right upper arm will rotate clockwise; your left upper arm will go counterclockwise.
5. Feel broad across your collarbones, like there's a smile spreading across your chest.

Tip: If your beach chair doesn't have armrests, for The Arms, step 2, squeeze your elbows into your lower rib cage.

About Flipper

Happy-Go-Yoga's Flipper deconstructs and puts a friendly spin on a yoga pose called Dolphin, which is basically Downward-Facing Dog on your forearms, or a prep for Forearm Stand (Pinchamayurasana: *PIN-chuh-MY-ur-AH-suh-nuh*). Together, they let you strengthen and stretch while you chill out. As you flex your feet and dig/drag your heels in the sand, you firm your core and leg muscles, from the thighs, to the calves, and even to your feet! Wrapping your upper arms into your body tones your arms, shoulders, and upper back while stretching the shoulders, neck, and chest. You'll be powered up for the ocean swim in no time!

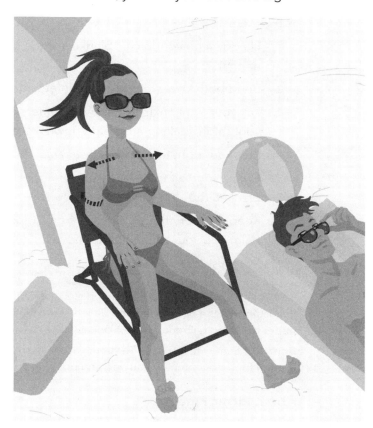

Picnic Pigeon

relax ▪ relieve

The grass looked really soft when you got to the park, and your picnic blanket is pretty comfy, too, but you've been sitting for quite some time and your back is stiff. To loosen up, you could get up and toss a Frisbee, or you could lie back and relax for relief, assuming you don't have to guard your food from eager pigeons.

Happy-Go-Yoga

1. Lie down on your picnic blanket (or the grass, if you really want to get earthy).
2. Bend both knees and press your feet into the blanket.
3. Lay your right ankle just above your left knee, where it starts to turn into your thigh, making an upside down 4 shape.
4. Flex your right toes toward your ankle.
5. Check yourself to make sure your upper back and your head are on the blanket, too.
6. Keeping everything where it is from steps 3 through 5, press your right palm into your right thigh to move it gently away from your face.
7. Switch sides.

Bonus A: To deepen the stretch, interlace your hands at the back of your thigh (hamstring) of the bottom leg and pull the entire 4 toward your face. Try to keep your upper back and tailbone on the blanket.

Bonus B: Start with Bonus A. To stretch a little more, make a bigger 4 by lifting the bottom foot, straightening your leg and pressing your foot on the sky.

About Picnic Pigeon

Sitting a long time is a fast track to lower-back stiffness, especially if you don't have any support. Picnic Pigeon is Happy-Go-Yoga's more relaxed take on the very popular hip opener Reclined Pigeon Pose. As you bring your ankle over your knee, you rotate and open up your hips by stretching out muscles that get tight from sitting and walking, including the piriformis and the gluteus muscles. It also helps create more suppleness in the iliotibial (IT) band, a band of tissue that can become tight as a rope and add to back stiffness. Flexing your toes helps protect your knee joints. So try Picnic Pigeon a few times during your picnic, 'cause back stiffness is no walk in the park!

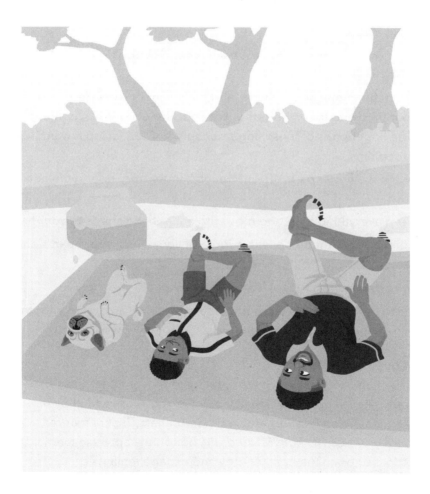

Love Multiplier

love • connect • inspire • brighten

Someone in your family is having a hard time, and there's not a lot you can do to help the situation directly. Rather than feel helpless, try sending more love, compassion, and positive vibes their way. At the same time, you'll expand your capacity for love in other ways, too.

Happy-Go-Yoga

1. Hold your palms so they face each other, but don't put your hands together.
2. Keep the thumb, index finger, and pinkie finger extended. Then, bend your third and fourth fingers at the knuckles and interlace/interlock them. (The finger pads of those fingers should now be facing inward, toward your palms.)
3. Touch the finger pads of your thumbs, index fingers, and pinkie fingers now.
4. Keep everything as is, and move the entire hand shape to your heart.
5. Connect your thumbs to the middle of your chest, your heart's energy center.
6. Gaze down and see the extra heart you hold in your hands.
7. Close the eyes, sit up tall, and breathe. Gaze inwardly with your thoughts into the heart for a few minutes (or as many as you'd like).

About Love Multiplier

Yogis make hand shapes, which are extensions of heart energies; they are, literally, shapes from the heart. Happy-Go-Yoga's Love Multiplier is a slight variation on Heart Energy mudra (Anahata Chakra mudra: *AHN-uh-HAH-tuh CHUH-kruh MOO-druh*), honoring Japanese martial arts practices to open the heart energy and expand feelings of compassion and love. It's said that as you bring more attention to that space and breathe a little deeper, this mudra can promote healing and also support lung and heart health. Our hands physically extend right from the chest, which holds the heart. When we make shapes or reach out, we broaden the reach of the feelings in our hearts. Think of a hug, blowing a kiss, petting a dog, or high-fiving someone to celebrate a moment of glee—those are love multipliers, too!

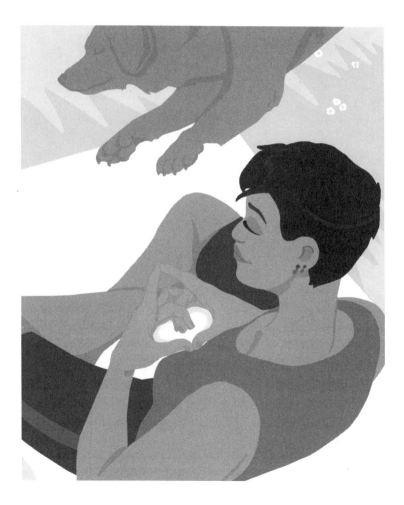

chapter eight

Crowd Control

Peaceful and powerful ways to cope with a crowd

One of the hardest things to do is stay calm and collected when you're in a crowd: You're getting jostled, dealing with people cutting in line, or even just plain bored waiting for the main event. For thousands of years, yogis have honed certain practices so that they can try to be the best of themselves no matter what's going on around them. Often, our patience and ability to remain calm are tested in big crowds when we can't control anything. So test out some of these Happy-Go-Yoga techniques when you're in the most challenging, crowded situations for ways to be steady despite chaos.

In this chapter:

Have a Seat ▪ **Shape Shift** ▪ **Happy Hipster** ▪ **Perched** ▪ **No U Di'n't**

Have a Seat

strengthen ▪ **focus** ▪ **balance**

I can't miss the pre-game show! Why isn't the stadium line moving? Redirect your frustration. Instead of hunting someone down to figure it out, build your strength and steady yourself mentally and physically, a mood that might be handy later…in case the team isn't doing as well as you'd hoped.

Happy-Go-Yoga

1.   Stand about twelve to sixteen inches away from a wall, with your back to the wall and your feet about hip width apart.

2.   Bend your knees and lean your upper body against the wall.

3.   As you bend your knees farther, walk your feet out more so your knees stay lined up above your ankles.

4.   Keep trying to melt your midsection toward your spine, and melt your spine into the wall.

5.   Inhale and prepare. Exhale and stay.

6.   Keep breathing!

7.   Imagine your tailbone is heavy as it descends down the wall (and try not to arch your upper back to lean back on the wall).

8.   Try to keep more weight in your heels to have an even balance of weight from the front to the back of your feet.

Bonus: Without a wall—do all the same steps, but lean your body forward a little bit at an angle as you sink your rear lower. You'll have to pay extra attention to steps 4, 5, 6, and 8.

Note: The without-a-wall version can look a bit like you're squatting in a not-so-pleasant Porta-Potty, but the good news is that Have a Seat might take you out of your head so much that you just don't care!

About Have a Seat

Happy-Go-Yoga's Have a Seat is based on a surprisingly hard pose in yoga, Chair Pose (Utkatasana: *OOT-kuh-TAH-suh-nuh*). Some yoga practices actually call this Awkward Pose (see Note for a little more info on just how awkward it can be). Have a Seat strengthens and tones the rear, as well as all the muscles in the legs. It also helps create stability in the knees and works your core as you keep it firm to support your back. Have a Seat is hard, so you'll be less distracted by other things, inspiring you to sit and be patient through the pose. You might need more of that if there's a delay in the game, too.

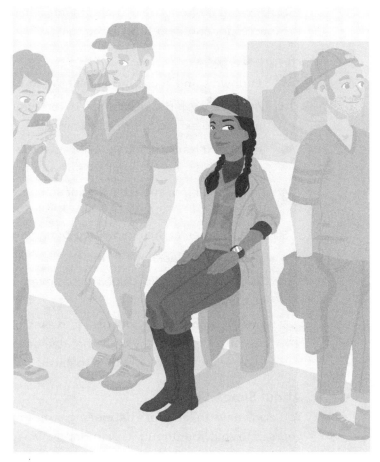

Shape Shift

focus ▪ **calm** ▪ **de-stress**

There's a big sale at the mall. Kids are running around. Frenetic bargain hunters are grabbing things and pushing people out of the way. It's mayhem all around you, and you're about to lose your mind. Take a minute, sit down, and shift back to balance again. You'll be in better mental shape to make your way through the masses for another round at the sale rack.

Happy-Go-Yoga

1. Sit down somewhere. It doesn't have to be a quiet spot.

2. Visualize a soft but vibrant ball of red energy at the base of your spine. Inhale and exhale calmly a few times.

3. In the next round of inhale/exhale, let the color of the energy ball shift to orange and move it to the area of your hips. Continue breathing.

4. Keep breathing, and let the color shift to yellow, right above your belly button.

5. Shift to green at the heart. Keep breathing smoothly.

6. Shift to light blue at the throat and lips. Inhale and exhale.

7. Shift to a deep indigo blue right above the center of your brows. Breathe in, breathe out.

8. Finally, let the energy dissolve into a violet lotus flower right above the top of your head. Stay there, breathe even deeper, and trust that you'll know when it's the right time to finish.

About Shape Shift

You don't have to let what's happening around you destroy your mood. Train yourself to shift your thoughts with Happy-Go-Yoga's Shape Shift and get your mind in shape for anything that comes your way. With practice and dedication, you can choose what to put in your mind. Shape Shift is a meditative mind exercise based on the system of the chakras (*CHUH-kruhz*), or subtle energies of the body that are said to support hormones and endocrine systems. The colors of the rainbow correspond to the chakras (think: ROYGBIV—red, orange, yellow, green, blue, indigo, violet), and the locations of the energies map back to areas of the physical body, creating the full spectrum of light. By imagining the shape, shifting the subtle energies of the body, you create lightness within you instead of feeling weighed down by frenzy. It's enlightening, to say the least!

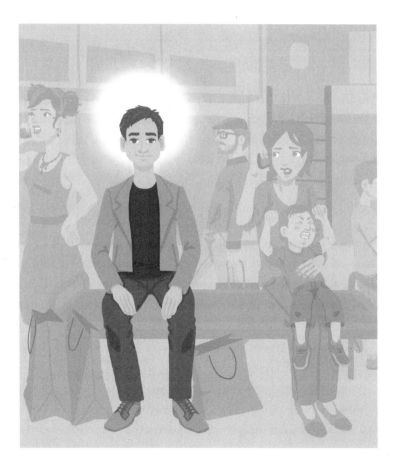

Happy Hipster

energized ▪ balance ▪ inspired

Standing in line at the checkout stand, you're bored, bored, bored. Turn a long wait into a practice of shifting your weight—and soon you'll be dancing your way to the front of the line. Hum your favorite tune in your mind or aloud.

Happy-Go-Yoga

1. As you stand in line, feel the weight of your body evenly between both sides of your body.

2. Keeping both feet on the ground, transfer your weight to one foot and leg, then, switch sides.

3. Lean to the first side again, letting your hip pop out in the direction of your lean, and direct your upper body to lean in the opposite direction,

4. Switch sides, and pop your other hip out while leaning your upper body in the opposite direction.

5. Keep going, maybe to a musical beat in your mind.

6. Let your hips groove as much as you'd like, swaying and leaning from side to side.

7. Repeat all steps as needed, desired, or inspired!

Extra Karma: If you keep doing this for several beats, it's inevitable that you'll be dancing in your own way. No one has to know what you're doing, but there's a good chance others will feel your vibe.

About Happy Hipster

Happy-Go-Yoga's Happy Hipster is inspired by the fun energies of the second chakra, Svadhisthana (*svah-dee-STAH-nuh*). I often call this the "fun" chakra, because it's related to playful exploration and sensuality. Physically, you stretch the outer hip and iliotibial band, which can sometimes be tight from a lot of sitting and standing. This pose also draws upon some of the basics of a pose called Standing Half Moon, which strengthens every muscle in the body's core and firms the waistline, rear end, and thighs. It also helps increase the flexibility of your spine. Whether you're a hipster or a hippie, you might discover everything is just groovy.

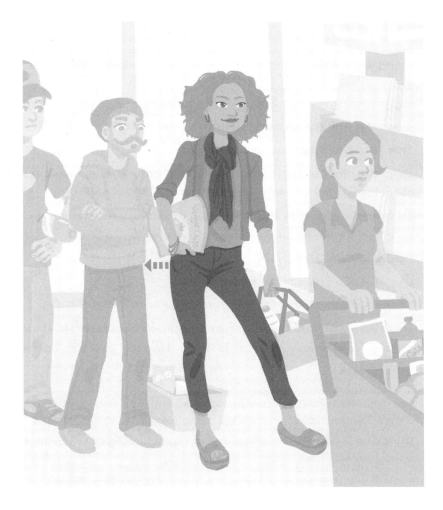

Perched

balance ▪ **strengthen**

Until your wait is over, use the time wisely to work on your balance—mental and physical—while strengthening your leg muscles ever so subtly. Like a bird, you're perched, ready to take action when it's your turn.

Happy-Go-Yoga

1. Stand with your feet together. Ideally, your big toes touch, but your heels are slightly apart.

2. Try to stand taller, but don't pinch your rear end together to do that. Press down through the ground instead.

3. Shift your weight to one foot and leg.

4. Bend the other leg to lift your foot off the ground, keeping your knees very close together and even touching.

5. Try to bend your knee more, keeping the knees together still, to bring your heel higher and closer to your rear end.

    Option A: Toes slightly off the ground

    Option B: Calf parallel to the ground

    Option C: Heel almost touching your rear end

6. Try to stay balanced for as long as you can by continuing to stand tall, drawing your tummy into your body, and firming your legs and rear end.

7. Switch sides.

Tip: If you try to lift the heel by using your muscles and not momentum, you'll find that Perched works better and will help you keep your balance!

Note: Don't do this in a moving vehicle unless you are holding on to something, and you are physically active regularly.

About Perched

Happy-Go-Yoga's Perched helps you find more balance, strength, and grace. Perched is based on a transitional pose in yoga to set up for a step back into a lunge. It helps keep the knees and hips aligned while activating the inner thigh muscles. Once in Perched, you'll stabilize your core and strengthen the standing leg's muscle while firming the rear end muscles of the lifted leg. When you align your hips and knees, you generally align the pelvis, which then helps arrange the spine for beneficial back posture. You can feel it on one foot, and even when you stand on both feet after finishing both sides of Perched. Ever notice that birds can stay perched on the smallest of places and still look graceful?

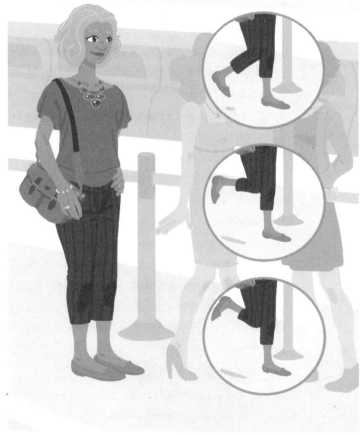

No U Di'n't

de-stress ▪ **empower** ▪ **strengthen**

Steam is coming out of your ears. You're dealing with too many obnoxious people—or is it you? Kids are running in circles. Have you just worn yourself into an angry place, with a packed schedule and no time to decompress? Use this ancient method to conquer bad vibes and burnout.

Happy-Go-Yoga

1. Wherever you are, find a space where you can reach your arms out to either side of your body without hitting someone.
2. Make a T shape with your arms, reaching firmly out from the shoulders.
3. Bend your wrists back so that your palms face outward and your fingers point upward.
4. Leave your index finger pointing up.
5. With the rest of your fingers, make fists and cross your thumbs over the fingers.
6. Keep reaching the arms out, relax your shoulders, and sit up as tall as you can.
7. Soften your eyes (but don't fully close them).
8. Make an O shape with your lips. Inhale so that the air passes over your tongue and feels cool
9. Close your mouth. Retain your breath without tensing up.
10. Exhale through your nose.
11. Repeat steps 6 through 10 for one minute to start, working up to three to five minutes.

Tip: For step 8, if you can, roll your tongue into the shape of a hot dog bun inside your mouth as you make the O shape. It creates a tubelike passageway for your inhale.

Bonus: To increase difficulty, extend length of pose to ten minutes (or more, if you're really angry).

About No U Di'n't

Happy-Go-Yoga's No U Di'n't is an attitude check, based on Suchi mudra (*SOO-chee MOOD-druh*), a gesture of inner cleansing, and an ancient Kundalini kriya (*KREE-yuh*), which is a yoga technique with a specific focus and goal. This one is meant to conquer inner anger and burn it out of your system. Yup. In No U Di'n't, your index finger represents the universe and possibly lessons learned with ease, while your thumb represents you and the fire element. Combined, the hand shape symbolizes your will to calm the inner inferno. As you extend your arms, you extend this energy from the center of yourself to the world around you (and perhaps enhance your personal space, to be honest). The breathing technique in No U Di'n't is called Cool Breath (Sitali Pranayama: *SHEE-tuh-lee PRAH-nuh-YAH-muh*), and is meant to reduce the internal temperature of your body. Just FYI, your shoulders will probably start to burn fairly quickly in this pose, but stay as calm as you can through the challenge…a metaphor for overcoming those moments that make you fume.

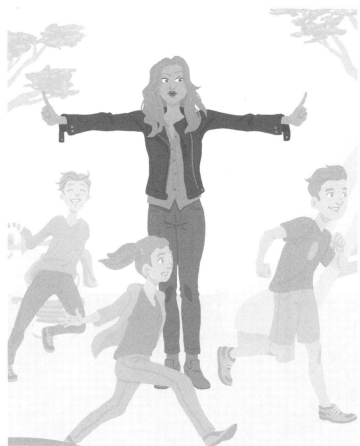

chapter nine

Happy-Plus-One

Significant (other) moments of love, connection, and tenderness

You can never get enough honest, pure love in your life. It's good for the heart, the soul, and your health! Countless studies have found that people in happy relationships have overall better health in several different ways. In fact, a Carnegie Mellon University study found they're less likely to get sick. Researchers at the State University of New York found that happily married people had the best blood pressure, and Ohio State University researchers found that people in positive relationships healed more quickly, physically. Other studies have linked long-lasting relationships to a longer life.

So, whether you're dating, have a life partner, are married, or just want to bring more za-za into the bedroom, here are a few Happy-Go-Yoga ways to invite more moments of love into your life with your significant other or another person of great, loving significance.

In this chapter:

Two for Devotion ▪ **Dinner and Dancing** ▪ **Lover's Lift** ▪ **Eternal Flame**
Snore Ignore ▪ **Soul Mates** ▪ **Pillow Talk** ▪ **We're Easy** ▪ **Joined** ▪ **One**

Two for Devotion

love ▪ connect ▪ calm ▪ inspire

Two hearts beating as one…that's really how you feel about each other. Sit close to each other and feel your devotion—hand in hand, heart to heart.

Happy-Go-Yoga

1. Sit next to your significant other, pretty closely. Your legs might even be touching.
2. Place your inside hands, the ones closest to each other, on your own heart energy centers (the center of your chests).
3. Feel your palms spread across the center of your chests (perhaps you start to feel a heartbeat).
4. Connect your outside palms, the ones farthest from each other, to each other.
5. Relax, especially at the shoulders, and breathe.
6. Close your eyes and feel the connection.

Tip: Try to keep that little space between your connected palms slightly open. with a bit of softness in the webbing of your hands and in your knuckles to prevent strain within the pose.

About Two for Devotion

There are fewer words in our language that describe the depths of the heart, like *devotion*. Just saying the word inspires feelings of deep love, commitment, and connection. Happy-Go-Yoga's Two for Devotion is a blend of one of the best-known expressions of devotion in all of yoga, Hand Gesture of Devotion (Anjali mudra: *AHN-juh-lee MOOD-ruh*) and a partner yoga technique. Your upper arm muscles, as you hold this pose, are challenged (sometimes you'll feel it in just a few minutes). At the same time, you'll give your hands, fingers, wrists, and arms some extra flexibility. Two for Devotion is a hand shape to show respect and a connection to each other's hearts. When you put your hands together, your hearts are brought together in a pure place, and you transfer more love to the other person with each breath.

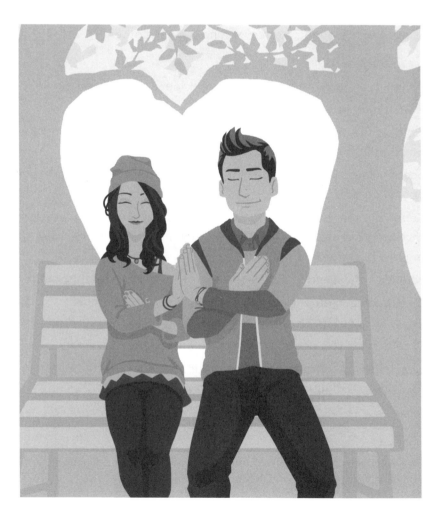

Dinner and Dancing

connect · focus · love

It's date night at that Mexican restaurant you've been dying to try, and one of you is texting and checking email (maybe both of you). Don't be that couple. Use this pose to disconnect from everyone but each other.

Happy-Go-Yoga

1. As you face each other, make sure your feet are solidly on the floor.
2. Switch phones with your person.
3. Holding the other person's phone, put both your hands behind your back with tops of your hands touching your back.
4. Scoot a little forward, so you're more toward the edge of your seat (but not falling off).
5. Keep your rear ends in your seats, and twist at the ribs so that your right shoulders are moving toward each other and your left shoulders are moving backward.
6. Feel your chest and heart space expand, from shoulder to shoulder.
7. Gaze into each other's eyes as you twist.
8. Match your breath here: Inhale a little more in the twist, and on the exhale, see if you both can twist more but still breathe easily.
9. Change sides, together, matching your breath as you move.
10. Repeat steps 5 through 8 on the other side.

Bonus A: Switch sides again if you want to keep dancing; you also don't have to start on the right side—either side is fine.

Bonus B: Keep each other's phones during dinner to keep your connection going over dinner conversation (yes, actual dinner conversation).

About Dinner and Dancing

Once upon a time, when couples made a date, they went on the date and talked to each other. Now, it seems couples are on the date but also chatting with everyone else on their phones. Happy-Go-Yoga's Dinner and Dancing gives you a way to get out of the phone and into a conversation by making the phone take a backseat (literally). You'll also loosen neck muscles and stretch the shoulders and chest. Your gaze helps you practice focusing on just one thing…the adorable person sitting across from you. Dinner and Dancing is a combination of a pose that opens the heart energies and twists the body called Rotated Triangle Pose (Parivṛtta Trikonasana: *puh-VRITT-tuh TREEK-oh-NAH-suh-nuh*), and the arm movements from the traditional Mexican Hat Dance (yes, that's what I said). Not only does Dinner and Dancing support a true connection on your date, but twisting can also help you digest. And, after you digest dessert, some real dancing might be in order, now that you've warmed up with the Mexican Hat Dance.

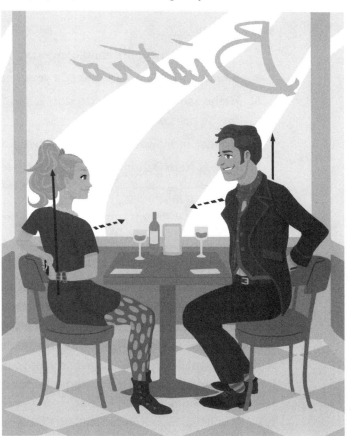

Lover's Lift

refresh ▪ love ▪ strengthen ▪ inspire ▪ balance

It's been such a long day that falling face-first into your pillow and into a deep sleep is your first desire, but your partner has that loving gaze. You realize you must rise to the occasion. Use this pose to refresh for *love*. (Or, use it anywhere you need a quick jolt of energy for something equally important!)

Happy-Go-Yoga

1. Face each other and stand comfortably in your socks or bare feet.
2. Inhale, and lift your arms above your heads, reaching high.
3. At the same time as you do step 2, lift your heels off the ground to balance on the balls of your feet.
4. Exhale, and lower your arms and heels at the same time.
5. Repeat steps 2 through 4 two more times, or more if you need more energy.

Bonus: On later repetitions, hold your inhale for a count of four as you balance on the balls of your feet with your arms lifted (you can expand to a six or eight count if you feel comfortable).

About Lover's Lift

We may not be diagnosed with chronic fatigue syndrome, but we've all been totally exhausted at times. Love doesn't have to suffer. Lover's Lift helps give you more energy on the spot, so the words "Not tonight, honey" don't come out of your mouth. It's Happy-Go-Yoga's version of Mountain Pose in the Viniyoga tradition, a small part of that practice's prescription to address actual chronic fatigue syndrome. You can do it together to strengthen your calves, ankles, and feet with the lift in the legs. Raising your arms helps open your chest for more breath, while taking more breath into your body helps feed it with refreshing oxygen. The arm motion also helps encourage blood flow throughout your body (yes, everywhere). After Lover's Lift, you should be a little more awake, so proceed…as desired.

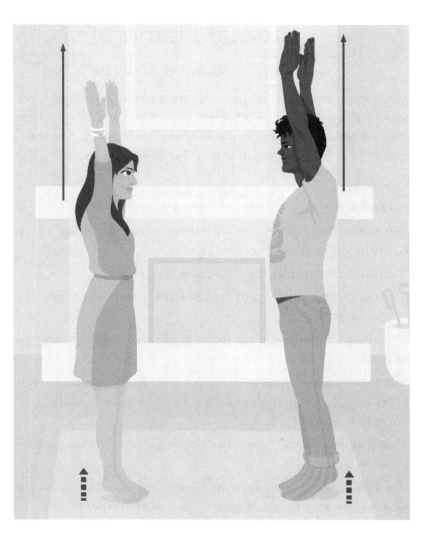

Eternal Flame

relax ▪ love ▪ connect ▪ focus ▪ calm

Even though you're hanging out by candlelight, and the stage is set for romance, you can't really get your mind off other things. Plus, you're a little tired, too. Use a candle flame to steady and clear your mind from the day's activities, then gaze at each other with full, loving attention and added eternal intimacy.

Happy-Go-Yoga

1. Darken the room.
2. Light a candle and place it on the floor or a low table safely, so it will be slightly below or at the level of your eyes.
3. Sit on the floor; use a cushion for comfort if you like.
4. Try to put slightly more than 1 yard of space (1 meter) between your gaze and the flame.
5. With your posture upright but relaxed, and your shoulders soft, gaze at the candle together.
6. Breathe normally and calmly for about thirty to sixty seconds; try not to chat or blink (you'll probably feel tears start to form, but resist blinking your eyes as long as possible).
7. Close your eyes gently. Stay quiet. You might have the candle's image still in your mind.
8. After a few breaths with your eyes closed, when the candle image goes away, reopen your eyes and gaze deeply, with a clear mind and soft heart, at your partner.
9. Repeat steps 5 through 8 twice more if you'd like.

Tip: It'll help to decide how long you want to do Eternal Flame before you start. Work together to create a shared signal to close your eyes in step 7 and open your eyes for the loving gaze in step 8. (An alarm is kind of a romance buzzkill, but if you do set one, choose some alluring or sweet sound as the ringer, please.)

Note: Remember to put out the candle flame safely.

About Eternal Flame

If the eyes are distracted, often the mind is, too. Eternal Flame is a variation of Trataka (*TRUH-tuh-kuh*), the concentrated gazing practice in Hatha yoga. Gazing at the candle helps you to focus, both physically and mentally, and holding steady to the point of tearing cleanses the eyes (think eyewash). Smooth breathing with soothing lighting can also calm and center you. Traditionally, this is done with a small oil lamp, which can be steadier than a candle, but a candle is fine, too. Eternal Flame can also be done as a cleansing practice for your mind, helping you detox from a busy day and be fully present for your significant other in that moment.

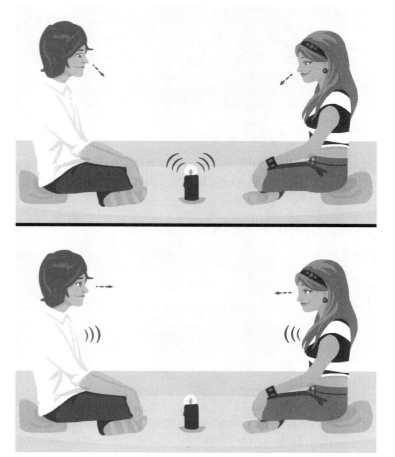

Snore Ignore

calm ▪ **relax** ▪ **relieve** ▪ **love**

The noise next to you is epic. You didn't realize such a snore could come from the same darling face that kisses you good night. It's keeping you awake, and you know that's not good news for the next day. To continue to feel loving toward this noisemaker next to you, you have no choice. You must Snore Ignore.

Happy-Go-Yoga

1. On your back, bring your knees close into your chest or press your feet into the bed so that your knees lift the covers.
2. Let your knees fall, together, toward your snoring person, and let your face look the other way.
3. Let your arms be open to the sides (above your shoulders or below, depending on room on the bed and your comfort), and have your palms face up to keep the chest open for breathing room.
4. Inhale fully and exhale fully.
5. Inhale through your nose more slowly and softly, and pause gently at the top of your breath without straining.
6. Exhale slowly through your nose to let your breath out (more like a content sigh, not a big, huffy sigh).
7. At the same time as in step 6, surrender to the twisting of your body, like you could sink into the bed.
8. Repeat three times, letting go and deepening your twist with each breath release.
9. Switch sides: send your knees to the other side and shift your gaze the other way.
10. Repeat steps 5 through 8.

Tip: If your back or shoulders get tight in the twist, use a pillow underneath your knees (as shown) to lessen the twist and get more comfortable.

About Snore Ignore

Snore Ignore is a combination of a reclined twist, Jathara Parivartanasana (*juh-TAR-uh par-EE-var-tuh-NAH-suh-nuh*), and a calming, stabilizing breath called Complete Method Breath (Sama Vritti Pranayama: *SAH-muh-VREE-tee*). Together, they help to turn on our internal quieting and calming systems when the real noise around you (aka epic snoring) is going strong. Snore Ignore's breathing helps soothe the nerves. As you twist, you gently release the worry that this noise will never end. If you do use a pillow, it can help encourage deeper reception of total relaxation, as in Restorative yoga, a type of yoga practice that reduces overstimulation and allows our bodies to release on a much more profound level. When your partner is in deep sleep, and the noise matches that intensity, Snore Ignore can be your own restful solution, so you are still inclined to call your s.o. "Darling" in the morning. The good news…at this point, at least someone is getting some sleep. And if all else fails…earplugs.

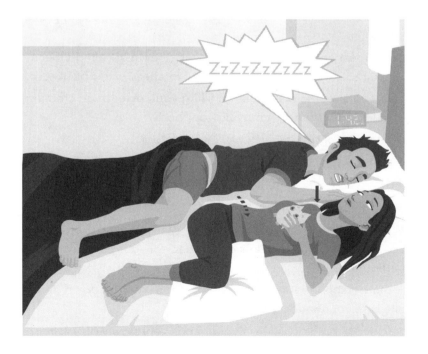

Soul Mates

relieve ▪ love ▪ connect ▪ de-stress

Your S.O. (significant other) is complaining of lower-back tightness. Nothing too serious, but you sure wish you could dissolve your beloved's discomfort. The longer it goes on, the more you feel your person's pain too. Perhaps your loving, healing hands can help—partner up for a little relief in the comfort of your home.

Happy-Go-Yoga

Give your person these directions:

1. On a soft surface, come to hands and knees, with your palms facing down, fingers pointing forward, and the tops of your feet on the floor.
2. Position your knees in one of two ways to ensure room to breathe:
   Option A: Directly under you so your shins are parallel
   Option B: Slightly wider so your shins make a V shape with your toes together
3. Sink your rear end back toward your heels (they might almost touch) and walk your hands farther forward. Support your forehead with a blanket or pillow.
4. Inhale and imagine that breath is filling your lower back, creating a dome-like effect, without moving your body.
5. Exhale and feel gravity relax you into the floor.
6. Keep breathing.

You do this:

1. Stand behind your person, near his or her toes.
2. Widen your feet to feel stable in your stance.
3. Place the heels of your palms on the back of your person's pelvis with your fingers toward you.
4. As your person breathes out in step 5, press straight down gently and make sure your hands don't slip!
5. After several breaths, release your hands very slowly (this is important).

Note: Step 5's slow release helps maintain the relief you just provided.

Note: If, at any point, your person is short of breath or feels discomfort in the knees and toes, have him or her come out of the pose for a hug instead. Also, skip this one if your person is a pregnant woman!

About Soul Mates

They say soul mates can feel each other's emotions and sensations even as they're in different bodies. If your partner is hurt, you can't help but feel a little hurt, too. You're that connected. Happy-Go-Yoga's Soul Mates enables you to help alleviate discomfort from one of the most common complaints in our world today: lower-back pain. As your partner takes Child's Pose, or Balasana (*buh-LAH-suh-nuh*), he or she is gently stretching the hips, thighs, and ankles while calming the brain and relieving stress. As you press down gently on the back of the pelvis, you encourage a lengthening and widening of the spine, which gives the vertebrae and discs some breathing room. Sometimes our upright ways (sitting, standing) can make things feel compressed and tight down there. Your palms can also be a gentle massage for your soul mate's lower-back muscles as you press down. Make sure you're calm too, because you want to transfer as much healing from your heart and hands as possible.

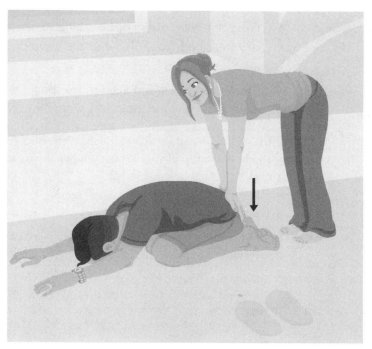

Pillow Talk

connect · **balance** · **relax** · **love** · **relieve**

Both of you have just flopped into bed, and it's the first chance you've gotten to connect all day long. Take some time to share what's going on with each other while finding some physical relief, too.

Happy-Go-Yoga

1. Lie on your sides together, facing each other.
2. Prop your heads up with your bottom hands, and try not to sink into your shoulders.
3. Keep your legs lengthened, or bend both knees slightly to help you balance on your side.
4. Firm your tummy without holding your breath.
5. Press the palm of the opposite hand into the bed space between the two of you to help you roll the upper shoulder open and create more room across the chest.
6. Breathe and imagine even more spaciousness across your chest, maybe even moving your shoulders wider and away from each other.

Bonus: Using the hand that was touching the bed, reach back, bend the knee of the top leg, and hold the top of your foot or your ankle. Try to keep your knee from lifting above hip level, then do this:

1. Keep the bottom knee bent for support.
2. Press the top of your foot or your ankle into your hand, away from you.
3. At the same time, imagine reaching the knee farther away from your top shoulder.
4. As you press your foot more, it should start to move away from your rear end.
5. Expand your heart and chest toward your S.O.

About Pillow Talk

There's a sense of closeness when you share intimate moments to wind down the day. Happy-Go-Yoga's Pillow Talk and its bonus version combine two yoga poses: Side-Reclining Pose (Anantasana; *AHN-un-TAH-suh-nuh*), and a variation of Half Moon Pose called Ardha Chandra Chapasana (*ARD-uh CHUN-druh chuh-PAHSS-uh-nuh*). As you firm your tummy, you strengthen your core by staying in the side balance. As you prop up your head with one hand and press into the bed with the other, you'll broaden across your collarbones. Breathing deeper, you open up the heart space and the ability to give and receive. In the Bonus version, by holding onto your foot or ankle and pressing backward with it, your shoulder opens up to reveal even more of your heart. The front of your hip and thigh get a stretch, too, which helps you let go of pent-up emotions. Now that you've let it all out with your trusted person, the pillow is right there so you can drift off to sleep together under a peaceful moon.

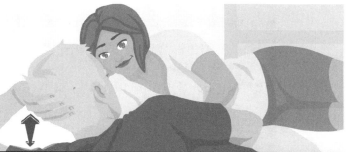

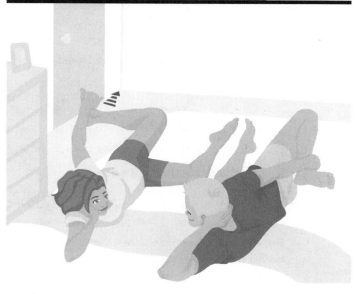

We're Easy

connect ▪ love ▪ calm

There's a little push-pull in every relationship, but we don't always know when we're pulling and when we're pushing. Make things easier on yourself and each other, by creating greater communication around the push-pull. Bind in yoga to bond with one another.

Happy-Go-Yoga

1. Make sure you are comfortable as you sit side by side in cross-legged seats.
2. Let your shins and feet relax. Leave space between your heels and your pelvis.
3. With the hand that is closest to the other person, cross at the forearms and place your palm on the other person's knee.
4. Wrap your other arm around your back by bending at the elbow and letting the back of the hand rest against your lower back, or even deeper, into the hip crease that is closest to your person.
5. Together, inhale, and sit up taller.
6. Together, exhale, and feel your chest expand as you move the front of your shoulders backward.
7. Inhale, and feel the other person sit up taller.
8. Exhale, and feel your heart stay lifted and open.

Tip: For more comfort, put a pillow or sofa cushion underneath your rear end or sit against the wall (with a little room for your arms to reach behind).

Bonus: As you continue to open your hearts, your shoulders might soften even more, giving you the room to reach farther behind you and hold hands with your partner, so you bond in front and in back.

About We're Easy

We're Easy is Happy-Go-Yoga's take on Sukhasana (*soo-KAH-suh-nuh*), or Easy Pose. On its own, this pose uses breathing and stillness in the shape to help calm your brain, strengthen your back, and stretch your knees and ankles. With the partner connection, you share the desire to help each other feel grounded, too. Add in the arm bind, and both of you get a stretch across your chest and shoulders, while your hearts are encouraged to be bigger, together. Yogis believe the ultimate peaceful and happy place is where we experience a balance of effort and ease in anything we do. As you take this pose together with your person, you might need to adjust and accommodate each other. At the same time, you help each other find ease…especially when in a bind. Isn't that what true partnership is all about?

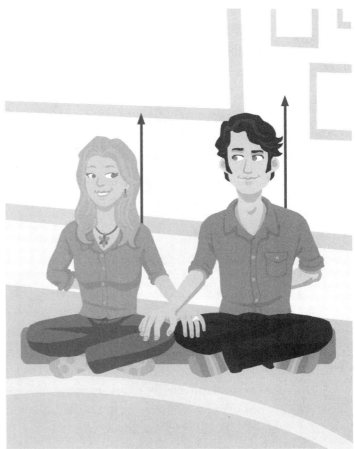

Joined

connect ▪ love ▪ relieve ▪ relax

Everyone says you two are joined at the hip. What if you were really joined at the hip to help each other relax and feel good, plus have each other's back at the same time?

Happy-Go-Yoga

1. Sit with your backs to one another, feet on the floor.
2. Link arms at the elbows.
3. Person A: Breathe in. Person B: Breathe out.
4. Person A: Breathe out and fold forward. Person B: Breathe in and lean back smoothly without lifting anything off the floor.
5. With the next breath, Person B: Breathe out and fold forward. Person A: Breathe in and lean back.
6. Keep breathing and seesawing your bodies as a unit, so your bodies and breathing are quite literally joined.

About Joined

In Happy-Go-Yoga's Joined, you combine a partner yoga version of Easy Pose or Sukhasana (*soo-KAH-suh-nuh*), the same one you did in We're Easy (p. 168). This time, you're arm-in-arm for the ride. When you lean forward, you'll strengthen your core and back muscles, and when your S.O. leans backward on you simultaneously, it's a nice stretch across the chest and shoulders. There's hip opening and spine alignment for both of you, too. When you switch, you return the favor to the other person. Seesawing back and forth in Joined helps couples use physical movement to create more awareness around how one person's actions affect the other — or, the push-pull effects of working and living together. Joined is Happy-Go-Yoga's way of helping us understand that joining forces and working together helps bring balance to both people in any situation.

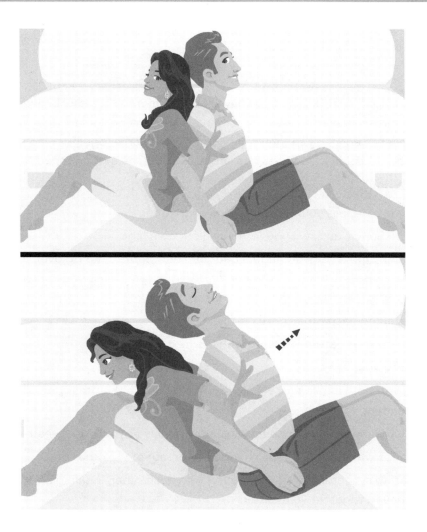

One

connect ▪ relax ▪ calm

It's been so long since either of you have had a moment to breathe. Between work, the kids, and everything else, quiet moments have become a total luxury. You don't have to plan an entire date night to steal some quality time together. Find just a few minutes to come together as one, and make this One moment special.

Happy-Go-Yoga

1. Sit down, cross your legs, and face each other.
2. Hold hands, and rest your arms on your own legs.
3. Slightly move your shoulders back, to keep from slumping over your heart. Instead, think of your heart getting bigger, filling your chest and sending love toward the other person.
4. Gaze into each other's eyes softly.
5. Soften your gaze even more with the next breath.
6. Close your eyes.
7. As you both inhale and exhale separately, notice the other person's breathing rhythm.
8. Bring a more calm, rhythmic, and slow quality to your own breath.
9. Notice whether that helps change the breath of the other person.
10. Start to synchronize your breathing with each other, inhaling and exhaling together with ease.
11. Open your eyes and gaze at each other again.

Note: You generally don't have to do this for very long, but you can do it for as long as you like.

Tip: To be more comfortable, you might choose to sit in chairs, or on a pillow or sofa cushion, as in We're Easy (p. 168).

About One

One is not a lonely number when your hearts are "as one." This Happy-Go-Yoga pose sets up a moment to really focus on one another. As you sit facing each other, automatically there's a connection…and your lives become one in this action. And, when you send positive feelings to another person, it creates a chain reaction of happiness, according to the National Institutes of Health. It's also very powerful and intimate to look at each other without saying a word. When you close your eyes, the relaxed breathing helps calm each other by consciously producing the body's natural relaxation response, which, according to many medical studies, can help lower blood pressure and reduce stress to boost life span. As you fine-tune this pose, you'll also fall into a rhythm with your S.O.'s breath, helping the energy flow more smoothly between the two of you…until your energy becomes One.

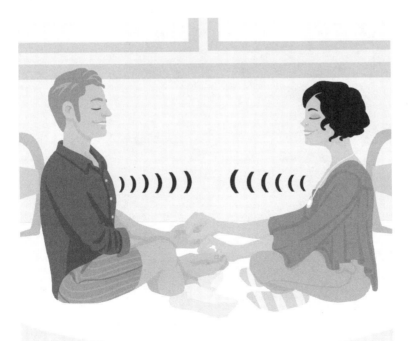

chapter ten

Global 24/7

Meditations to calm and inspire—anytime, anywhere

Each time I travel or explore somewhere new, I get brand-new perspective, because I leave my comfort zone. Yoga helps you explore places within your body and mind that you don't normally visit. This chapter is dedicated to the more mindful, quiet, and meditative side of yoga that is truly for anyone, anywhere, anytime.

The ancient yogis knew it, but now modern doctors are on board with mindful meditation—more than ever before. A recent study from Massachusetts General Hospital, the original and largest teaching hospital for Harvard Medical School, found that in just eight weeks, these mind-quieting practices made measurable changes in the brain regions associated with memory, sense of self, empathy, and stress, which can help improve our well-being and quality of life. These five universal Happy-Go-Yoga practices can really be done in any situation. The more you do them, the more you help yourself to yoga's greatest benefits: mental clarity, the ability to recognize happiness within, and inspiration to live your life to the fullest.

Keep exploring.

In this chapter:

Free Your Mind ▪ **The Snag** ▪ **Pause and Proceed**
Not So Ho-Hum ▪ **Make a Change**

Free Your Mind

relax · calm · balance

The rude person in the latte line this morning was just the beginning. Ever since then, people have been getting on your nerves or getting in your way. Time to free yourself from the frustrating clutter in your head with a meditation practice that helps clear clouds from your mind.

Happy-Go-Yoga

1. Inhale deeply, open your mouth, and let out a big sigh.

2. Visualize actual clouds in your mind.

3. Start to breathe deeply in and out through your nose, inhaling and exhaling evenly, without gasping for breath or sighing heavily.

4. Draw your focus to a single cloud. Inhale.

5. Exhale, and imagine your breath creating a soft breeze that pushes the cloud aside, out of the field of vision in your mind's eye, as if the cloud were one of your frustrations. (If you're really frustrated, one cloud might be stubborn and require a few extra breaths.)

6. Repeat steps 4 and 5, letting individual clouds drift away one by one.

7. With each cloud that clears, take a moment to notice the beauty and clarity of the blue sky in its place.

Tip: Your mind might begin to wander during this meditation. If it does, try not to get frustrated and create more clouds. Do your best to calmly come back to your breath and continue visualizing more blue sky in your mind, instead.

About Free Your Mind

As you imagine the clouds appearing in your mind and gently passing by with each breath, you allow thoughts to arise and dissolve, rather than allow those thoughts to remain and fester for self-created stress. (It's a little bit like that old saying, "This too shall pass.")

Happy-Go-Yoga's Free Your Mind is also an important yogic practice from the *Yoga Sutras of Patanjali* (*SOO-truhz of puh-TAHN-juh-lee*), the written philosophy that guides many types of yoga practices. One of the early sutras, setting forth the intent of yoga, is *Yoga citta vritti nirodha* (*YO-gush-EE-tuh VREE-tee nee-ROH-duh-huh*), which means: to stop the fluctuations of the mind, or calm the vibrations of the mind that cloud our ability to see clearly; to not react, and instead act from the best of ourselves, which usually emerges when we give ourselves space. If that means not getting worked up by the irritating guy in the latte line, and being able to reduce stress on my own, sign me up for a double shot of that.

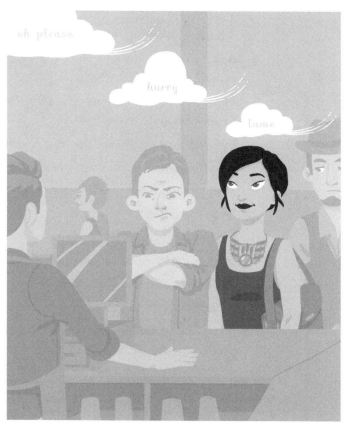

The Snag

de-stress ▪ empower ▪ strengthen

This problem you've been having is standing in the way of everything and seems as immovable as a stubborn elephant. Embrace the obstacle. As they say, sometimes things happen for a reason! Use The Snag to empower yourself for whatever happens next. Sometimes challenge can illuminate a totally different path.

Happy-Go-Yoga

1. Standing or sitting, bring your arms to a T shape, at shoulder height.
2. Bend your elbows, keeping them shoulder height, and bring your hands right in front of your heart.
3. Flip your left palm to face away from you, with the back of the hand close to your heart.
4. Flip your right palm to face toward your chest.
5. Join the palms, opposite fingers to opposite wrists.
6. Start to slide the palms apart in this position.
7. Snag the fingers in a grip.
8. Inhale, and tighten the snag.
9. Exhale, and slightly loosen the snag.
10. Repeat steps 8 and 9 a few times and start to feel tension dissolve.
11. When you start to feel a release, prepare to finish The Snag.
12. When ready: Inhale, tense your grip, then exhale, letting your fingers slowly release and move away from one another.

Tip: Keep your elbows shoulder height and out to the sides, and try to keep your shoulders from rising and creating tension in your upper body.

About The Snag

The Snag is a yogic hand shape called Ganesha mudra (*guh-NESH-uh MOOD-ruh*), inspired by the Hindu elephant-headed deity, Ganesha. He is the remover of obstacles that stand in your way, but he sometimes places obstacles in your path to guide you in a different direction, for a reason. Happy-Go-Yoga's The Snag helps you practice releasing tension intentionally. Roadblocks in life will always arise, but you can rise to the occasion and move beyond the snag that seems to be in your way. Meanwhile, you'll strengthen your shoulders, chest muscles, and hands while stretching your wrists. Holding hands at the heart helps circulation and keeps the blood flowing (not boiling) with the courage to face your obstacle. Now, you can move through it or head in a new, creative direction.

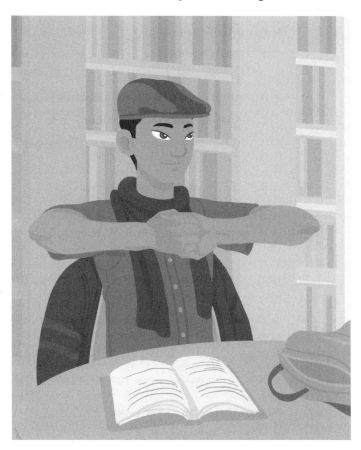

Pause and Proceed

calm · focus

You're overscheduled and rushing around; life is a blur. You find you're losing things, forgetting things, and even dropping things. Time to implement a personal pause before you proceed, so you can collect your thoughts and give your full attention to what you need to do.

Happy-Go-Yoga

1. Either sitting or standing, inhale normally. Notice if you're breathing quickly, and try to slow down your breath.

2. Inhale, exhale, and let all the air out.

3. Inhale while counting slowly to four.

4. At the top of your breath, with relaxed shoulders, suspend your breath for two counts.

5. Exhale while counting slowly to six.

6. Inhale normally, and exhale normally.

7. Repeat steps 3 through 6.

Tip: If you feel strain, stress, or light-headedness as you suspend your breath, reduce the suspension time. Keep practicing, and build up to longer periods of suspending the breath. Remember to count slowly.

Bonus: The more you practice this, the easier it will become. Work up to these counting patterns:

Inhale six seconds; suspend four seconds; exhale eight seconds

Inhale eight seconds; suspend six seconds; exhale ten seconds

About Pause and Proceed

When life gets so busy that you don't remember what you did a few minutes ago, it's time to slow down. Happy-Go-Yoga's Pause and Proceed helps remind you how to shift from the fast-moving treadmill of life to appreciate individual moments that make up your life. Based on yoga's breathing technique kumbhaka (*KOOM-buh-kuh*), or retaining the breath, Pause and Proceed asks you to take a deliberate pause in the inhale-exhale cycle, putting you in control of giving yourself permission—and a valid reason—to pause. There is a moment of doing nothing—neither inhaling nor exhaling. Over time, the practice of giving yourself a "nothing" moment will help you feel less pressure to do the next thing on your list as quickly as you can, because you trust that it will come, even if you pause. That, in turn, helps give you more clarity to actually move on to the next thing, feeling secure, calm and focused. On those days you think you don't have a moment to breathe, take a moment to put a pause in your breath—and then proceed with a clearer mind.

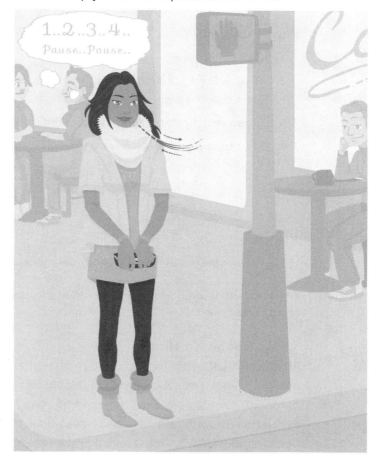

Not So Ho-Hum

balance ▪ inspire

You feel nothing can pull you out of these blahs, but you really want to snap out of it. If you're uninspired, unmotivated, and uninterested in almost everything but procrastinating, try repeating this simple phrase to get your mind and spirit going in a productive direction again—from "ho-hum" to "oh yeah"!

Happy-Go-Yoga

1. Close your eyes.
2. Take a deep breath in through your nose, open up your mouth, and exhale with a sigh.
3. Close your lips and begin to breathe normally.
4. Start to say, either out loud or in your mind:

   Not

   So

   Ho

   Hum

5. Repeat step 4 at least three times—more, if your blahs have a capital B.

Tip: I recommend you sit somewhere where you can close your eyes. It'll help you pay attention to the words without being distracted by what's going on around you.

About Not So Ho-Hum

Mantras (*MAHN-truhz*) are spiritual phrases that can empower, inspire, heal, and guide in the context of real life. Not So Ho-Hum is Happy-Go-Yoga's take on one of yoga's most powerful mantras, "Om hum, so hum." With no literal translation (though *So hum* translates to "I am that"), this mantra combines energy and breath to help elevate and awaken your state of mind as you stay connected to the rest of the world. As you say it, you may feel a teeter-totter kind of energy as the words make a sound pattern (either aloud or in your mind), which helps you to balance and unite the opposite energies within yourself. By changing the words to Not So Ho-Hum, Happy-Go-Yoga gives this ancient mantra a whimsical, but potent and modern spin that is relevant to that ho-hum feeling you might have every now and then. Not So Ho-Hum keeps it *real* and gives you a *real* way to try to beat the blahs right here, right now.

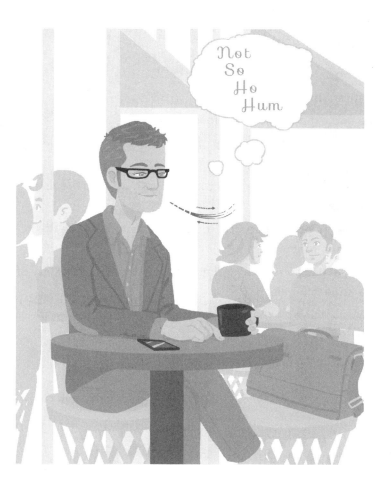

Make a Change

calm ▪ relax ▪ empower ▪ inspire

You feel stuck. You would like to make a change, but you're not sure. Sometimes, you're scared that change might not be good, but a small voice inside keeps telling you that if you take that first step, your life could go in a brand-new direction. This is some scary stuff. Start by inspiring yourself. Let go of something that no longer serves your desire to grow, and make room for new energy. It's in your destiny.

Happy-Go-Yoga

1. Sit comfortably.
2. Inhale and exhale normally a few times.
3. Close your eyes; lay the backs of both hands on your knees with your palms facing up. Inhale.
4. Say "Saaa" as you exhale, and touch your thumbs to the tips of your index fingers. Inhale.
5. Say "Taaa" as you exhale, and touch your thumbs to the tips of your third fingers. Inhale.
6. Say "Naaa" as you exhale, and touch your thumbs to the tips of your fourth fingers. Inhale.
7. Say "Maaa" as you exhale, and touch your thumbs to the tips of your pinkie fingers.
8. Repeat steps 4 through 7.

Tip: This meditation and chant are usually done for twelve minutes. Try to start with a few rounds, then work up to it. Don't worry if your first attempts don't last long. It takes practice!

Bonus: You might decide to say this mantra in your mind at first, but as you feel more comfortable, work up to this:

First round: spoken aloud

Second round: at a whisper

Third round: quietly in the mind

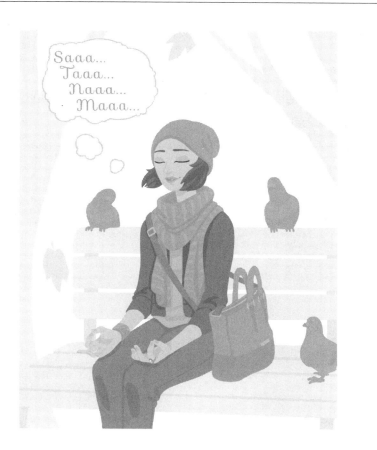

About Make a Change

When you repeat this spiritual phrase, it's said you flood your mind with happy neurochemicals. At the same time, it's believed to boost your intuition, balance the hemispheres of the brain, and spark a catalyst for change by connecting your mind, body, and spirit to the cycle of life. Make a Change in Happy-Go-Yoga is a blend of one of Kundalini yoga's original practices and the symbolism of the hands in the chakras (*CHUH-kruhz*) system, the subtle energies of the self. Touching the thumb to the tip of any finger is said to bring energies and elements into balance. There are several interpretations of the finger-element connection, but in this take, your thumb represents the transformative fire energy within.

Tap it to your…

Index finger to balance your love and compassion (Sa = infinity).

Third finger to balance your self-expression and creativity (Ta = life).

Fourth finger to balance your foundation and roots (Na = death).

Pinkie finger to balance your emotions and relationships (Ma = rebirth).

There are days when change seems impossible, but trust that, with each breath, the potential for change is in your hands. You can shape your destiny.

sources

introduction:

How I Got Happy: The Author's Story
Concept: mind helps the body, body helps the mind; Timothy McCall, M.D., "The Science of Yoga," chap. 2 in *Yoga as Medicine* (New York: Bantam Books, 2007).

chapter one:

Who, Why, and How to Happy-Go-Yoga

UCLA Study
"Mindful Awareness Can Reduce Stress and Anxiety; Ease Depression and Pain," UCLA Health, November 8, 2013.

University of Illinois
Diana Yates, "A 20-Minute Bout of Yoga Stimulates Brain Function Immediately After," University of Illinois News Bureau, June 5, 2013.

Duke
Meera Balasubramaniam, Shirley Telles, and P. Murali Doraiswamy, "Yoga on Our Minds: A Systematic Review of Yoga for Neuropsychiatric Disorders," abstract, *Frontiers in Psychiatry*, January 25, 2013.

Taiwanese Research
Chin-Ming Jeng, Tzu-Chieh Cheng, Ching-Huei Kung, and Hue-Chen Hsu, "Yoga and Disc Degenerative Disease in Cervical and Lumbar Spine: An MR Imaging-Based Case Control Study," abstract, *European Spine Journal*, August 15, 2010.

chapter two:

Travel Buddies

Chapter Introduction
Christine Chen. "Suffering from Presidential Stress?" MSN Healthy Living, *The Daily Apple Blog*, November 5, 2012.

Eagle Perch
Based on classic Garudasana, p. 97; B. K. S. Iyengar, *Light on Yoga* (London, England; Harper Collins UK, 2009).

Eagle Twist
Classic yoga twist, no source.

Bird's Eye
Based on classic Kundalini eye exercises.

Bird of Prey
Classic yoga arm bind, no source.

Hang Time
Adaptation of classic Bakasana (Crane or Crow Pose). P. 315; "Light on Yoga," Iyengar, *Light on Yoga*.

Grounded in a Good Way
Adaptation of classic Vrksasana (Tree Pose), p. 62; Iyengar, *Light on Yoga*.

Reach for the Moon
Adaptation of Bikram Standing Half Moon Pose; Bikram Yoga College of India; with adaptations via Viniyoga style.

Walk Your Puppies
Popular movement in Downward-Facing Dog, no source.

Pray to the Seat Pocket
Adaptation of preparation for forearm stand, with "prayer" hands. No official name, no official pose, commonly used throughout yoga practices.

Smooth Landing
Adaptation of Nadi Shodhana (Alternate Nostril Breath) p. 445; Iyengar, *Light on Yoga*.

chapter three:
Career Counselors

Wrist Wrestling
Personal practice.

Confidence Booster
Christine Chen. "Can You Fake It 'Til You Make It?" MSN Healthy Living, *Daily Apple Blog*.

Twist, Don't Shout
Classic yoga seated twist, no source.

Total Brain Power
Hakini mudra; Gertrud Hirschi, *Mudras: Yoga in Your Hands*, (New Delhi: Sri Satguru Publications, 2000) p. 112.

Stand Your Ground
Classic Pada Bandha, no source.

Let It Roll
Personal practice.

Spine Align
Adaptation of Restorative yoga (as learned in the tradition provided by Judith Hanson Lasater).

Forgive the Frenemy
Mushti mudra; Pushpaputa mudra; Hirschi, *Mudras: Yoga in Your Hands*, pp. 106, 164.

Counter Pose
Classic adaptation of Pigeon Pose, standing use.

Office Warrior
Supported Warrior III classic, no source.

chapter four:
Road Rage Relief

Car Kali
Traditional deity/mythical story of Goddess Kali; pose created by Dana Flynn and Jasmine Tarkeshi, cofounders of Laughing Lotus Yoga Center in New York City.

Nimble Warrior
Classic hand movement in Warrior flow series, Christine Chen Yoga adaptation.

Road Hips
IT stretch: commonly known, adapted by Christine Chen Yoga.

Rearview Mirror
Classic yoga teaching on relaxing the face to communicate to the brain; supplemented by concepts in *The Yoga Face*, Annelise Hagen, (New York: Penguin, 2007).

Unlock Gridlock
Alignment based on Iyengar, *Light on Yoga*, p. 71; Urdhva Drishti: David Life, "The Eye of the Beholder," *Yoga Journal*.

Road Warrior I
Own Warrior I practice with a block; based on the story of the warrior struggle in the Bhagavad Gita—general theme of the critical chapter of the Mahabharata.

Road Warrior II
Classic yoga pose with multiple trainings.

Get Toe'd
Variation on Utthita Hasta Padangustasana: Iyengar, *Light on Yoga*, p. 77–78; "Orthopaedic Surgery Sports Medicine Guide to Cracking and Popping," Johns Hopkins Medicine.

Parking Karma
Thanissaro Bhikkhu, *Noble Strategy: Essays on the Buddhist Path* (Distributed by Metta Forest Monastery 1999).

Hey DJ
Ayurveda principles, personal practice.

chapter five:
Chill, Homies

Dive Right In
Personal practice.

Dish It
Uddiyana Bandha; simple modification from *Yoga Journal* and Iyengar, *Light on Yoga*.

Surf It
Skandasana; different in the disciplines; using Vinyasa tradition.

Garden with the Gods
Vajrasana; Srivatsa Ramaswami, *The Complete Book of Vinyasa Yoga*, p. 177–178 (New York, Da Capo, 2005).

Laundry Lift
Utkata Konasana/Goddess Pose; Yoga Basics.

Superhero
Iyengar, *Light on Yoga*, pages 120 & 176.

Towel Glide
Personal practice.

Smartphone Siesta
Salamba Sirsasana; *Yoga Journal* sample version; Brahmari Breath.

Couch Potato
Classic Viparita Karani.

X-tra R&R
Classic Yin Pose.

chapter six:
Sunny-Side Up

Shine On
Variation on classic Surya Namaskar, common practice.

Wise Dreamer
Classic yoga teaching on relaxing the face to communicate to the brain; and adaptations from Hagen, *The Yoga Face*.

Flap and Fly
Kundalini kriya, classic practice.

***V* is for Verve**
Prasarita Padottanasana, classic pose.

Brush and Breathe
Sama Vritti, Iyengar, *Light on Yoga*, p. 453.

Rock Your Heart
Seated Cat-Cow, used as a classic warm-up and reduced Camel Pose (Ustrasana), Iyengar, *Light on Yoga*, 87.

Sunshine Coffee
Bhastrika breath: Chopra Center.

Unbreakable You
Vajrapradama mudra, Unshakeable Confidence and Trust; Hirschi, *Mudras: Yoga in Your Hands* p. 160.

Swimmingly
Fish Pose variation, Matsyasana; Iyengar, *Light on Yoga*, p. 138.

Simba
Lion's Breath, Simhasana; Iyengar, *Light on Yoga*,
p. 135.

chapter seven:
Family Fun

Slither
Based on classic Bhujangasana; Iyengar, *Light on
Yoga*, p. 107.

Jaws
Sternocleidomastoid; Ray Long, *The Key Muscles
of Yoga*: Scientific Keys, vol. I, (Bhanda Yoga:
2007) p. 197.

Mind the Monkey
Mudgara mudra: Cain Carroll and Revital Carroll,
Mudras of India, p. 160; Timothy McCall, *Yoga as
Medicine*; traditional story of the Ramayana.

What-EVER!
Personal practice; Long, *Key Muscles of Yoga*,
p. 157–160.

Sprout
Adaptation of Vikasitakamalasana (Blossoming
Lotus Pose); "Blossom and Grow," *Yoga Journal*,
and Sharon Gannon, "Blossoming Lotus,"
Jivamukti Yoga, June 2006.

Hug of Joy
Combination of Laughing Lotus's Breath of Joy,
Sama Vritti Pranayama, and Hatha yoga Breath of
Joy, from Yoga International.

Through the Fire
Agnistambhasana; "Fire Log Pose,"
Yoga Journal.

Flipper
Dolphin Pose preparation for Pincha Mayurasana
(Feathered Peacock Pose or Forearm Stand).

Picnic Pigeon
Reclined pigeon pose; adaptation and variation
on the common One-Legged King Pigeon Pose.

Love Multiplier
Anahata Chakra mudra: Carroll and Carroll,
Mudras of India, p. 42; Christine Chen, "Every-
day Shapes from the Heart," ChristineChen
Yoga.com blog post.

chapter eight:
Crowd Control

Have a Seat
Utkatasana (Chair Pose) variations p.88; Iyengar,
Light on Yoga.

Shape Shift
Universal chakras system.

Happy Hipster
Standing Half Moon; "Half Moon Pose," Bikram
Yoga.

Perched
Basic move to step back to a lunge; personal
practice.

No U Di'n't
Kundalini kriya; Sochi mudra; Hirschi, *Mudras:
Yoga in Your Hands*, p. 104–105.

chapter nine:
Happy-Plus-One

Chapter Intro
Sherry Ruah, "10 Surprising Health Benefits
of Love," Medicine.net, 2009.

Two for Devotion
Anjali; Carroll and Carroll, *Mudras of India*,
p. 44; practice tip from "Salutation Seal,"
Yoga Journal.

Dinner and Dancing
Personal practice: classic Rotated Triangle Pose and Mexican Hat Dance.

Lover's Lift
McCall, *Yoga as Medicine*, p. 249. (chronic fatigue treatment sequence.)

Eternal Flame
Trataka, *Hatha Yoga Pradipika* and Yoga Bible/ Cleansing Kriyas, Candle Gazing, p. 344 (Great Britain, Godsfield Press, 2003).

Snore Ignore
Reclined version of Jathara Parivartanasana (Stomach-Revolving Spinal Twist) and Sama Vritti Pranayama.

Soul Mates
Child's Pose standard teacher assist; also see "Child's Pose, *Yoga Journal*.

Pillow Talk
Classic poses; "Peak Form," *Yoga Journal*, and "Side-Reclining Leg Lift," *Yoga Journal*.

We're Easy
Classic Sukhasana pose.

Joined
Classic Sukhasana partner variation.

One
National Center for Complementary and Alternative Medicine, "Relaxation Techniques for Health: An Introduction," National Institutes of Health, February 2013, and "Stress Management Health Center," WebMD, National Institutes of Health, "Happiness Spreads Through Social Groups."

chapter ten:
Global 24/7

Chapter Intro
"Mindfulness Meditation Training Changes Brain in 8 Weeks," news release, Massachusetts General Hospital, January 21, 2011.

Free Your Mind
Buddhist meditation.

The Snag
Ganesha mudra; Hirschi, *Mudras: Yoga in Your Hands*, p. 60.

Pause and Proceed
Kumbhaka breath; adapted from various sources, including Sharon Gannon and David Life, *Jivamukti Yoga* (New York: Ballantine Books, 2002) p. 106.

Not So Ho-Hum
Thomas Ashley-Farrand, *Healing Mantras* (New York: Ballantine Books, 1999) p. 165.

Make a Change
Kundalini yoga/Kirtan kriya; Carroll and Carroll, *Mudras of India*, p. 30; Hirschi, *Mudras: Yoga in Your Hands*, p. 31.

acknowledgments

Thank you to my Mom, Dad and family, who taught me health is everything; to my close friends who stood by me through the daily ups and downs; to my careful doctors who listened closely when I told them something else needed to happen; to my patient and compassionate teachers who kept me optimistic that something good keeps happening with each breath; to my students who continue to show up and transform right before my eyes.

Special thanks to my literary lookout crew: Bridget, Adam, Amanda and Libby...and especially to my husband, Richard, for believing I can do anything—anytime, anywhere.

– Christine

index

Christine Chen is an Emmy award-winning news anchor/reporter, wellness writer and editor, multi-certified yoga teacher, and former Athleta-sponsored athlete. Years ago, she began squeezing yoga classes into her hectic schedule, desperate to de-stress from a high-intensity job and ease a back condition that left her in non-stop pain. Yoga not only worked, but it transformed her life forever. Today, she finds great joy in sharing her fun, practical yogic approach to feel better and be happier in a busy, busy world. A San Francisco native, Christine lives with her husband in New York, where yoga helps her live a life of wellness—anytime, anywhere. For more information, visit www.happygoyoga.com.